'When we read Alys' account of the experience of having Covid-19, and also her treatment in hospital, we were in no doubt that we wanted to include it on our Tales of Lockdown blog. Alys' lucid prose gives the reader a real sense of the disease – and has you hanging on the edge of your seat, willing her to pull through! I would strongly recommend it to anyone if they are in any doubt as to the huge impact of the virus on physical and mental health.'

Polly Wright, Artistic Director of The Hearth Centre

'This is an honest and emotional account of the realities of having Covid-19. It illustrates clearly not only the physical impact but the trauma and emotional impact too. This is hugely relatable if you have been through this, and a moving insight if you haven't. It shows how the committed care of others, personal strength and hope make recovery possible.'

Claire, Counsellor, Mind Conwy

# WARD NINE:
## CORONAVIRUS

Alys Morgan grew up in the West Midlands, and like many people from that area, has English, Welsh and Irish ancestry. She is a retired teacher and librarian who lives in north Wales, and enjoys reading, writing and walking. A survivor of Covid-19, she considers she owes everything to NHS Wales and Mind, who cured her body and soul. This book is a love letter to both of them.

Dr Pyrke lives in Cardiff and has worked in hospitals across south Wales. He is currently an Internal Medicine Trainee working in the second wave of the pandemic.

*Ten percent of the cost of this book will be donated to Conwy Mind in helping them to support those, like Alys, who continue to be affected by the pandemic.*

# WARD NINE: CORONAVIRUS

One Woman's Story

Alys Morgan

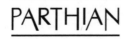

Parthian, Cardigan SA43 1ED
www.parthianbooks.com
First published in 2020
©Alys Morgan 2020
ISBN 978-1-913640-31-6 paperback
Editor Kathryn Tann
Cover design by Jeremy Simon
Cover image: iStock
Typeset by Elaine Sharples
Printed by 4Edge Limited
Published with the financial support of the Books Council of Wales
British Library Cataloguing in Publication Data
A cataloguing record for this book is available from
the British Library.

Earlier versions of this book first appeared as diary excerpts,
online, as part of The Hearth Centre's *Tales of Lockdown* project
(www.talesoflockdown.org).

*Dedicated to NHS Wales, who cured my body, and Conwy Mind, who cured my soul.*

*In memory, also, of all those who have died at the hands of this virus, without their loved-ones by their sides. They will not be forgotten.*

*A dreadful plague in London was*
*In the year sixty-five,*
*Which swept an hundred thousand souls*
*Away; yet I alive!*

Daniel Defoe, *A Journal of the Plague Year* (1722)

# FOREWORD

In late December 2019 a cluster of atypical pneumonia cases of unknown cause were formally reported in Wuhan, China. The location common to this cluster was a 'wet' seafood market in the same city. Fast-forward a month and on the 30th January 2020, the World Health Organisation labelled this novel strain of Coronavirus, now christened COVID-19, a cause for international concern.

The news of this new concern permeated the hospital wards in half-understood news articles. Every conversation became a series of unanswered questions: How deadly? How infectious? How would we keep patients safe? We were busy to breaking point already – *how could more be done*? The stories and images from China, Italy and Spain brought new worries. The major fear unspoken, but widely understood, was that we as doctors may have to become unfeeling triaging machines, dealing out ventilators to a select few. The thought was terrifying.

Then, as time passed, the hospital changed. People came together; plans were put in place and whole systems of working restructured. The National Health Service is a cumbersome juggernaut but once it changes direction and puts its mind to something, it does it well. Intensive care bed capacity doubled; staff were trained to do completely new tasks and whenever their help was needed, willing volunteers from every department – from cleaners to nurses, catering staff to doctors – flooded forward.

Treating someone with COVID-19 is scary. Doctors and nurses are accustomed to feeling in charge, but with COVID-19 there is very little control. In the early days there was no meaningful treatment. We could give supportive care: an intravenous drip, anti-sickness medications, painkillers, oxygen and, at a last resort, being put to sleep and mechanically ventilated. All these things buy time but none of them actively treat the virus. The patient must get better on their own.

To see a patient on oxygen struggling to breathe, and to know how little you can offer, feels like failure. These aren't numbers in a political briefing. It's you and a patient in an alien room – and they are unwell, terrified and alone. We should never forget that this is about people. We shouldn't forget that it's about our NHS.

On 11th March 2020, COVID-19 was declared a global pandemic – and everything was going to change.

Dr B. Pyrke, Junior Doctor, NHS Wales

One Woman's Story

I was drifting slowly down a tunnel. It was more grey than black, and there were sparkling lights floating in it. I could hear the voices of Mom and Dad calling to me, and I was quite happy. I went on towards the lights.

There's truth in those stories we hear about what it's like to brush close with death. There was light as well as dark. And there wasn't any fear.

I came back to consciousness with a start. There was a light, but it was the glaring overhead light of Ward Nine. I was in my hospital bed, and being held up and forward. Somebody – a man in full PPE – was kneeling behind me on the bed. There were sharp blows on my back, and his fists were closed in front of me, in what I recognised as the Heimlich manoeuvre. I knew this from First Aid courses at work, but I'd never expected to see it in action.

I was choking, and then it all came up, into the basin that Nurse Susan was holding in front of me.

Later, when the nurses had changed my gown and all the bedsheets, Susan came over.

'You stopped breathing,' she said. 'We called for the doctor, and when he came, he said you were choking on your own vomit in your sleep.'

I'd spent the last part of two weeks being constantly sick; now, apparently, it had nearly killed me.

1

Susan came closer.

'You need to *try*,' she said gently. 'You need to *try* so you can get better. Please *try* for me. And all of us.'

I closed my eyes.

'Sue,' I said at last, 'I honestly don't care anymore. If I could close my eyes and just drift away, I would. I think I actually want to die. I can't stand it any longer.'

I opened my eyes. She was staring at me, and I think there were tears in her eyes.

# PART ONE

*It was about the beginning of September, 1664, that I, among the rest of my neighbours, heard in ordinary discourse that the plague was returned again in Holland ... We had no such thing as printed newspapers in those days to spread rumours and reports of things, and to improve them by the invention of men, as I have lived to see practised since ... But it seems that the Government had a true account of it, and several councils were held about ways to prevent its coming over; but all was kept very private.*
(Daniel Defoe, *A Journal of the Plague Year*)

## Saturday March 21<sup>st</sup>

And so they always say that you remember where you were when you first heard of it.

Mom used to say:

'I was playing in the back yard when war was declared. Dad came out, and sat me on his knee and told me about it. I thought nothing of it.'

Went to the library today and was just browsing when Jane, one of the library staff, came over.

'Borrow as many books as you want,' she said, looking distressed. 'We've just had a call. We close at noon today and we don't know when we will open again.'

I watched as she went round telling everybody – she didn't make an announcement. I think it was to stop people from panicking.

I gathered up a stack of paperbacks from new books and returned books, and as I checked them out, Tash, the other library assistant, told me about the digital book download service. Not sure I can master that.

I've never known public libraries to close before. I was working in Birmingham libraries when the city centre was bombed back in 1974. The next day we all went back in as normal, and every library opened. I remember the caretakers were standing in front of a table as we went in, and they said, 'Check your bags, please.' It was the first time I had ever heard that phrase, which I was to hear for the next twenty years.

Mom started work during the war, in munitions, and she went in every day. When the sirens went off, she said, they used just to put on their tin hats and carry on working. In the evening she went to the pictures, usually the Lozells Picture Theatre. One night she decided to go to the Youth Club at Burlington Hall instead. That night, the picture theatre took a direct hit and everyone was killed.

4

*Surely never city, at least of this bulk and magnitude, was taken in a condition so perfectly unprepared for such a dreadful visitation … They were, indeed, as if they had had no warning, no expectation, no apprehensions, and consequently the least provision imaginable was made for it in a public way.* (Defoe)

## Sunday March 22nd

Johnson was on TV but I didn't watch it. Can't stand the way his hair always needs brushing. My dad worked in a factory for fifty years and never turned up looking like that. Brylcreem, and when he couldn't afford it water, but always immaculately brushed. Followed it on the BBC Live blog. Apparently we are now in lockdown, though nobody quite knows what that means and as far as I know I'm in work tomorrow. A furlough scheme has been announced for those who cannot work, and some of those would not otherwise have been paid.

So what is lockdown? I thought of Mom talking about drawing the curtains for a blackout for the very first time. And curfews. I had a look on the BBC website to see what exactly we *can* do. We can take one form of exercise a day, so I will walk down to the beach (the spring weather is beautiful). We can shop for basic and essential goods (no more trips to M&S for party clothes). Travel is permitted for essential work. Our local cinemas and theatres have already closed, and now pubs and restaurants must close their doors too. As must caravan and camping sites, and B&Bs, hostels and hotels. This is a terrible blow to our local tourist industry. Looking at the *Daily Post* website, I saw that many of our banks and post offices are reducing their hours. There was also a list of which essential services can remain open, including garages, petrol stations – and bicycle shops (so we can all exercise, and cycle to work!).

People are saying that these are the most significant set of restrictions to be imposed on this country since World War II (and already reports of people breaching them).

> *Let any one who is acquainted with what multi-*
> *tudes of people get their daily bread in this city by*
> *their labour, whether artificers or mere workmen—*
> *I say, let any man consider what must be the*
> *miserable condition of this town if, on a sudden,*
> *they should be all turned out of employment, that*
> *labour should cease, and wages for work be no*
> *more.* (Defoe)

I looked up pictures of the Coronavirus on the internet. It is a round ball, with spikes sticking out of it, and looks rather like a sputnik. I stared at it some time. I don't fancy that rolling about in my body. It is of course the kind of thing that happens to other people.

## Monday March 23$^{rd}$

First day back in work in the new lockdown. Very quiet in the college library. First thing I noticed when I came in today was a hand-wash dispenser presumably put up over the weekend, and Mary the receptionist had put a line of supplies in front of her desk. She gave me some gloves and a hand wash.

Lots of rumours sweeping the site; we're part of a much bigger college complex. I heard that we might close on Tuesday.

Lots of frantic last-minute arrangements about contacting staff and students via Google Meet. The library at the main site had set up last-minute training sessions on this. Decided to close the library early and go to one at 4pm.

I caught the bus as I'm trying to avoid driving, because of my arthritis, although it suddenly struck me that I was safer driving – travelling in my own car. At Colwyn Bay a poor old man got on, carrying a box and a carrier bag. He didn't seem well at all. I heard him chatting to the bus driver as he fiddled for change.

'Got thrown out at two hours' notice,' he said. 'I'm on my way to Llandudno to find a shop door to sleep in.'

I remembered hearing that homeless people living in branches of a national hotel chain had been thrown out as the hotels closed down.

I got out my purse, and gave him some money.

'Go to the police,' I said, though I didn't hold out much hope of anybody being able to help him.


*Beggars.*
*'Forasmuch as nothing is more complained of than the multitude of rogues and wandering beggars that swarm in every place about the city … It is therefore now ordered, that such constables, and others whom this matter may any way concern, take special care that no wandering beggars be suffered in the streets of this city in any fashion or manner whatsoever, upon the penalty provided by the law, to be duly and severely executed upon them'.* (Defoe)


Arrived at 3.30pm to find the library staff assembled. Philip, the librarian, had called an impromptu staff meeting.

'We're all closing at five o' clock today,' he said. 'You will all be working from home. You can take a laptop home if you need it, and I'll be setting up staff meetings on Google Meet.'

I was relieved I'd come over to the training meeting set today, which was the first and last. So now I know how to use Google Meet.

Thought about the poor old man tonight, and wondered if he'd found anywhere to sleep.

## Tuesday March 24th

First day of working at home. I can't say it's my first experience of home working, as I had to take a few days off during the petrol strike in 1999. I didn't have the internet then so I seem to remember taking masses of files home with me. Catrin was nine so I didn't have to entertain her too much; it must be hard for people with small children.

So it's all online now. I checked the library email regularly and sent round an email to staff and students offering help with any catalogue and information services. I had my NVQ folders to work on, which are all online. But I can't see my students finishing this summer, and I don't think I'll be finishing my Internal Assessors' award either.

Huge shortages in the supermarkets as people stockpile. Rumours of people escaping to holiday homes, an option most of us don't have.

*On the other hand, many that thus got away had retreats to go to and other houses, where they locked themselves up and kept hid till the plague was over; and many families, foreseeing the approach of the distemper, laid up stores of provisions sufficient for their whole families, and shut themselves up, and that so entirely that they were neither seen or heard of till the infection was quite ceased, and then came abroad sound and well.* (Defoe)

## Wednesday March 25th

Caught the bus into Llandudno to get some book vouchers for birthday presents at Waterstones. Noticed that many of the shops on the High St were already closed, with sad notices up in their windows. And Waterstones was closing at 6pm as well.

Said, 'See you on the other side,' to the nice staff, but that sounded a bit final, really.

On the bus going home, noticed we all sat in separate seats. But people do that anyway, don't they?

On the news, deserted city centres. Eerie.

*Business led me out sometimes to the other end of the town, even when the sickness was chiefly there; and as the thing was new to me, as well as to everybody else, it was a most surprising thing to see those streets which were usually so thronged now grown desolate.* (Defoe)

## Thursday March 26th

Went with John to our local supermarket, Tesco. Overnight, they've made a lane to queue in, made up of trolleys on their sides – and slung between them was the yellow tape which they usually use to mark spillages.

We shuffled along with only so many people being allowed to go in at a time. I was quite relieved to see so many people, because sometimes I feel as if I've woken up into *The Day of the Triffids*.

A one way system was in place, and they'd put footsteps in all the aisles where you were supposed to go but we still ended up making mistakes. Bit irritating to go round all the supermarket.

Some of the staff were wearing masks and gloves.

The High St in Abergele was deserted, with all the non-essential shops closed. I felt sorry for the charity shops, and all the causes they support. And for the people who worked in our cafes and pubs and restaurants – all that low-paid work, relying on the whims of managers to survive.

## Friday March 27th

It helps that the weather is beautiful. Had my allotted hour of exercise as I've done every day this week. I walk down to the beach and along the coast path. Lots of cyclists out. I don't miss getting the car out at all.

Emails from our two local theatres, saying some shows we had booked to go to were obviously now cancelled. We could apply for a refund, or we could choose to count it as a donation.

It's a bad time for the arts. I thought about all the young people who would now be out of work. I've had so many good years going to the theatre, cinema, opera and ballet. And they are all something that cheers people up. There are, apparently, going to be a lot of live streams.

*All the plays and interludes ... were forbid to act; the gaming-tables, public dancing-rooms, and music-houses ... were shut up and suppressed ... for the minds of the people were agitated with other things, and a kind of sadness and horror at these things sat upon the countenances even of the common people. Death was before their eyes, and everybody began to think of their graves, not of mirth and diversions.* (Defoe)

## Saturday March 28th

Couldn't face the supermarket and its queues so I went down our little High St in Abergele. Some of the shops were closed, but I got meat at the butcher's, and vegetables and eggs at the grocer's next door. Both of them practising what they now call social distancing – they're such small shops that only one person can go in at a time, and hand wash is provided on the way in.

Bread at the baker's, and then I crossed over to our little Health Shop, which I use anyway. No problem here with hand wash or soap, she had plenty and all environmentally friendly. Also nice biscuits and tinned food.

Came back via Mr Patel's Convenience Store, where I picked up sanitary towels for Catrin and a few other things like air freshener.

Milkman had been when I got back. Left flyer saying that in addition to milk, he can provide salad and vegetable boxes, fresh juice, cream, sacks of potatoes, cheese and yoghurts.

Struck me that I'd done all my shopping without setting foot in the supermarket. The supermarkets are doing a great job, but it reminded me of the days when Liz and I used to go shopping with Mom in the small shops on Lozells Rd in Birmingham.

I feel like Mrs Miniver, or as if I'm living the *Diary of a Provincial Lady,* which should sound cosy and comforting, but isn't.

The BBC News is about nothing but Coronavirus. It's as though all our lives were leading just up to this point, and what went before didn't matter.

## Sunday March 29th

Worried about Catrin who lives in a housing association flat in Rhyl. She has a heart condition but she hasn't had a shielding letter, and as she works in a hardware store, she has to go in as usual.

John said he would do some shopping for her and leave it just inside the door; she can look in and pick it up.

I assume this lockdown means you can't see members of your own family. Liz phones every day; she's absolutely paranoid about getting CV. She can't see her sons or her grandsons. Something else that's different from Mom's accounts of the war, when the family all stuck together and refused to be evacuated. I can see this is going to make a lot of people very depressed.

> *We continued in these hopes for a few days, but it was but for a few, for the people were no more to be deceived thus … nay, it quickly appeared that the infection had spread itself beyond all hopes of abatement.* (Defoe)

## Monday March 30th

Enjoyed my walk, as always, along the coast path.

Continued my working at home by beginning a list of lockdown novels. Defoe's *A Journal of the Plague Year* and Samuel Pepys's *Diary* were obvious ones, as is Camus' *The Plague* (apparently a best seller on Amazon). I started thinking as well of books about being isolated – *Robinson Crusoe* and anything by Anita Brookner. And Jean Rhys.

All the schools are closed, of course. And there is not much evidence of children round here doing home learning. They are running around screaming while their parents sit drinking and barbecuing. At some point, the parents also start screaming. One thing the kids are learning is the use of the F word.

I don't ever remember the schools closing in my childhood, even for snow. Dad was at school every day in the Blitz. He said he was ecstatic when he turned up one morning, and the school had been bombed flat in the night.

Liz and I had a bit of home learning with Mom before we went to school. Mom could add things up in her head; she'd always finished her bill before the Co-op cashier rang it up. Her secondary school wanted her to go to Aston Technical College and do book-keeping, but she had to go to work in the Jewellery Quarter making munitions, because she was the eldest and her father had died at Dunkirk. They needed the money; Nan used to have to pawn her wedding ring every Friday for food, and beg for parish relief.

Mom hated reading and hadn't read a book since she

left school at fourteen, but she taught us to read using alphabet cards, and to count using an abacus.

Curious incident in the evening. I was sitting watching television when I heard the door open and close. Went out and saw Catrin, come to pick up her shopping. She obviously had a cold; her nose and eyes were streaming.

I said, 'Cat, surely you aren't at work?'

'Yes, I am, Mum, we're short staffed.'

'But they know about your heart?'

'I haven't had a shielding letter, Mum. So they say I have to be in.'

Went through a lot of emotions in thirty seconds; I couldn't send her away, looking like that. My natural instinct was to look after her. Reason told me I should not. What a dilemma for a parent.

'You know, you should go up to your room here and stay there. Your stepfather will phone them in the morning.'

I think she was quite grateful for this, but John looked concerned when I told him.

'I think lockdown means she shouldn't be here.'

A very difficult situation. I was reminded of something I had read in Defoe. A mother and daughter.

> ... *a certain lady had an only daughter, a young maiden about nineteen years old ... about two hours after they came home the young lady complained she was not well; in a quarter of an hour more she vomited and had a violent pain in her head. 'Pray God', says her mother, in a terrible fright, 'my child has not the distemper!'... While the bed was airing the mother undressed the young woman, and just as she was laid down in the bed, she, looking upon her body with a candle, immediately discovered the fatal tokens on the inside of her thighs. Her mother, not being able to contain herself, threw down her candle and shrieked out in such a frightful manner that it was enough to place horror upon the stoutest heart in the world ... As to the young maiden, she was a dead corpse from that moment, for the gangrene which occasions the spots had spread [over] her whole body, and she died in less than two hours.*

I suppose reading that story was the first time I really realised that any of us could die.

## Tuesday March 31st

Put my head round the door into Catrin's room. She was lying in bed, a hankie to her mouth.

'Don't come near me!'

Left a tray outside her room. She doesn't want to eat, so I left a jug of water, orange juice and paracetamol.

Went in quest of paracetamol, which took much of the day. None in any of the supermarkets. I ended up queuing at the chemist's, which is tiny, and we shuffled along, as only one person at a time can go in.

John watches the daily press conferences at 5pm, but I don't. I've noticed a lot of repeats beginning to appear on TV. Thank God for the radio and box sets.

It's not knowing the symptoms that makes it so difficult.

*And this is the reason why it is impossible in a visitation to prevent the spreading of the plague by the utmost human vigilance: viz., that it is impossible to know the infected people from the sound, or that the infected people should perfectly know themselves … people have it when they know it not, and that they likewise give it to others when they know not that they have it themselves; and in this case shutting up the well or removing the sick will not do it, unless they can go back and shut up all those that the sick had conversed with, even before they knew themselves to be sick, and none knows how far to carry that back, or where to stop; for none knows when or where or how they may have received the infection, or from whom … (Defoe)*

## Wednesday April 1st

Left a tray for Catrin with all the usual on and some tissues. I did wonder if she only has a cold or if it is CV. But she has no breathing problems, and doesn't seem to have a temperature. She is being sick.

As I was due to go for a hearing check at the doctor's, walked up to the health centre. The appointment was at 10am, and I got there for 9.45, feeling quite pleased I'd done my bit for the environment by walking.

Lots of confused people standing around the main doors, which were locked. We could see people at the desk, but nobody took any notice of us.

We walked around the building and eventually found a small door. It had a notice on it asking us to ring the bell if we had an appointment, so I did.

It was answered by a man in what I suppose is Personal Protective Equipment, or PPE. It's one of those new terms I've learnt, like social distancing or herd immunity.

He reared back in horror when he saw us standing there.

'Don't come any closer!'

I suppose it was like this in the times of the Great Plague and the Black Death and so on.

> ... *there were very few physicians which cared to stir abroad to sick houses, and very many of the most eminent of the faculty were dead, as well as the surgeons also; for now it was indeed a dismal time, and for about a month together, not taking any notice of the bills of mortality, I believe there did not die less than 1500 or 1700 a day, one day with another.* (Defoe)

A group of us were standing there, and we did what the British always do: we formed an orderly queue, and shuffled along, till we could get to the front and explain just why we were there. In a very polite fashion. When I got to the front, he stood some distance from me. I couldn't help imagining him wearing one of those Great Plague masks which look like a bird's beak. As it was, I could see nothing of his face. I explained about my clinic, and he said all clinics had been cancelled till further notice, and I should have had a text or call.

Went home feeling rather disappointed, because this appointment had seemed important to me and now it suddenly wasn't important. John said his diabetes clinic was also cancelled. It made me wonder about really important things, like chemotherapy, and all those NHS services we had always taken for granted. And also whether more people might die now those services were taken away.

## Thursday April 2nd

John had to take a bucket up to Catrin as she is being sick and can no longer manage the rush to the bathroom. I'm not sure that sickness is a symptom of CV.

I decided that she needed a doctor, and maybe she would get a home visit from somebody in full PPE. I called and to my surprise they answered straight away, but took our phone number and said it would be a telephone consultation only. I said in that case they needed her mobile number as she is in bed.

The doctor did ring within an hour, and diagnosed gastroenteritis. She prescribed something which she said would go straight to the chemist.

In the meantime, I gave her a Lemsip as she is still streaming. John is not sure whether she should register with something called NHS 100. Because she hasn't been diagnosed, she hasn't been tested, and as soon as we register with it, we are marked.

*Notice to be given of the Sickness.*
*'The master of every house, as soon as any one in his house complaineth … shall give knowledge thereof to the examiner of health within two hours after the said sign shall appear…'* (Defoe)

John went for the prescription later. He had to queue at the chemist's; there, they went in two at a time. I asked him to get paracetamol. It wasn't on display; they got it from under the counter and said it was being rationed to one pack per person. Well, we haven't got *formal* rationing, but people are fighting in supermarkets over soap, handwash and loo rolls.

Some neighbours taking advantage of being at home and are out barbecuing, with people there who are definitely not family.

*Feasting prohibited.*
*'That all public feasting, and particularly by the companies of this city, and dinners at taverns, ale-houses, and other places of common entertainment, be forborne...'*

*Tippling-houses.*
*'That disorderly tippling in taverns, ale-houses, coffee-houses, and cellars be severely looked unto, as the common sin of this time and greatest occasion of dispersing the plague ...'* (Defoe)

## Friday April 3rd

Catrin a bit better today. She drank a cup of tea and ate some grapes.

John thinks we need to switch to home delivery of food as she has been ill while here. We don't in fact know what she has been ill with; she had a telephone diagnosis, and nobody has actually seen her. The symptoms she has are not really those you read about on the NHS 100 Covid website (which I have just discovered). But he thinks we should be doing something called self-isolation and shielding; still all new terms to me.

In fact, the milkman can deliver much of what we need. I called in at the vegetable shop, the butcher and the health shop on the High St, and they also agreed to deliver; you order over the phone and pay by card, and they leave it on the doorstep later that same day. Liz was in a queue for a supermarket, and it was a three-week wait for delivery.

I wondered how older people who don't use the internet are managing. There was something in the free newspaper about the Council setting up a phone befriending service for older people, and that council staff working from home would deliver supplies. Also that our local food banks are now making home deliveries, and very busy. I thought I should really do some form of volunteering.

On Facebook, the nice deli I use in Colwyn Bay was also offering to do home delivery.

None of these places charged for delivery. I have

always used them and will continue to do so after all this is over.

It is said the police are turning people back at the Wales-England border.

> *This hurry, I say, continued some weeks, that is to say, all the month of May and June, and the more because it was rumoured that an order of the Government was to be issued out to place turnpikes and barriers on the road to prevent people travelling.*
> (Defoe)

## Saturday April 4th

Catrin had some toast for breakfast, and soup for lunch, and ate plenty of grapes. She thinks she may go home.

I did our telephone order for home deliveries. They ring the bell when they come, and leave your order on the doorstep. It's lovely bringing the boxes into the kitchen and sorting through them. I had a fruit, salad and vegetable delivery from the milkman, and it's all fresh and local.

Went on a walk down to the beach. Sat on a bench looking at the sea on the coastal path. It was a beautiful day, blue sky, blue sea, seagulls calling, cyclists whizzing down the cycle path. Everybody who passed me crossed to the other side of the path.

I suppose our lives are indeed like those who went through the war. A huge cataclysmic change in everyday life. Mom used to talk about this. Dad was evacuated and didn't think much of it. He said he'd rather have stayed in Birmingham, which he was used to, and that the thought of air raids was very exciting for a child. He found the countryside dull, and would rather have been in the thick of it (although it's lucky he wasn't, as his street took a direct hit).

But our situation is different in some respects. Mom still went out to work every day, even though Birmingham was being blitzed, while many of us are now off work (and missing the companionship). Mom was in the midst of all her family, apart from Grandad, who never came back from Dunkirk. And she did go out every night, whereas we have nowhere to go. We have to stay at home. Mom said it was going to jolly, bouncy American musicals, usually starring Betty Grable or Judy Garland, which got her through the war. We have no cinema at all. We are separated from those we love. We don't have any jolly, bouncy propaganda, just news which is full of doom and gloom.

When I got home, Catrin was well enough to have dinner, and said she is going back to the flat. John's main complaint was about getting cat food and cat litter for the cats; it's something our deliveries don't cover.

Record numbers of people signing on for Universal Credit.

## Sunday April 5th

Catrin went home. John says we must self-isolate now. Unclean, unclean.

> *Inmates.*
> *'That where several inmates are in one and the same house, and any person in that house happens to be infected, no other person or family of such house shall be suffered to remove him or themselves ...'*
> (Defoe)

The churches all closed for worship. Sad for those who want spiritual solace. Apparently, organisations such as the Samaritans and Mind are working flat out, dealing with people with depression and anxiety.

John tried to contact the box offices of the local theatre, where we had tickets for the film *Emma,* but there was an out of the office reply. I wonder how many theatres will reopen. Or shops, cafes, restaurants. Or if life will ever be normal again. People are talking now about the New Normal.

Mom used to say that in 1945 there was a sense of optimism – with a new government, the end of the war,

the welfare state to look forward to, Birmingham to be
rebuilt.

And maybe when this is all over – and who knows how
long it may go on? – we may be able to rebuild society,
in the model of the New Normal. But I don't feel
optimistic about the situation we are in. And I really
worry about the jobs situation. Thousands of job losses
are announced daily on the BBC – and there may not
be much for them to go back to. I'm close to
retirement; but what a sad time to be a young person.
So many of the students at my college are studying
things like Performing Arts or Hospitality or Hair and
Beauty; what a terrible outlook for them. My sister Liz
says the only certain employment at present is as an
undertaker.

*All families retrenched their living as much as pos-
sible ... so that an innumerable multitude of
footmen, serving-men, shopkeepers, journeymen,
merchants' bookkeepers ... and especially poor
maid-servants, were turned off ... These might be
said to perish not by the infection itself but by the
consequence of it; indeed, namely, by hunger and
distress and the want of all things: being without
lodging, without money, without friends, without
means to get their bread, or without anyone to give
it them.* (Defoe)

## Monday April 6th

Worked from home, on shared documents on the Google Drive. I've been at work forty years, and it's odd how things have changed. We're also doing an online enquiry service for staff and students, and of course they've got access to e-books.

Having read all my library books, I registered for the online books download service, although I struggled with the software.

Liz called later, or rather did something called Face Time, which she had to explain to me. It was nice to see her, although the phone screen is quite small.

She explained that she has been furloughed – understandably. It's not thought that catering staff can work from home.

My eldest nephew is working from home, as he's in computers. The youngest works for McDonald's and is furloughed. The middle nephew works at the Welsh Mountain Zoo, and he's in, because of course animals have to be looked after. Liz said the zoo is worried about their future financially though. Dreadful stories that animals in zoos may have to be destroyed. I promised to make a donation.

It was announced on TV that Boris Johnson had gone into hospital.

Food banks are very busy indeed.

> *However, the poor people could not lay up provisions, and there was a necessity that they must go to market to buy, and others to send servants or their children; and as this was a necessity which renewed itself daily, it brought abundance of unsound people to the markets, and a great many that went thither sound brought death home with them.* (Defoe)

## Tuesday April 7th

We had a staff meeting via Google Meet, something else I've had to master. Really, I would have liked to retire when I was sixty, but of course I didn't get my state pension. I have to go on till I am sixty-six. My works pension is tiny. You couldn't live, or even survive on it, despite forty years in local government and further education. I had to reduce my hours, first for Catrin's care when she was little, and later Mom and Dad when they were old and ill. So the occupational pension I received at sixty was reduced accordingly.

I just feel that things are passing me by now – I've reached the end of my learning curve, and don't want to learn any more about ICT.

Though it is nice to email friends, which I did in the

evening. Felt tired and went to bed early. Missed out on my walk.

Coronavirus seems especially rampant in the cities, where I grew up. Where people are crowded, and where people quite simply have to continue to go to work. And because so many of them do low-paid and now essential work.

> *It must be confessed that though the plague was chiefly among the poor, yet were the poor the most venturous and fearless of it, and went about their employment with a sort of brutal courage … scarce did they use any caution, but ran into any business which they could get employment in, though it was the most hazardous.* (Defoe)

## Wednesday April 8th

Awoke with a bit of a sniffle and was glad that I was not working from home. I have now finished until after Easter, and was relieved about that.

Didn't feel like coffee, and drank tea all day. Felt listless, as I always do with a cold, and did not go for a walk. I wondered if I had Catrin's bug, and looked at her prescription to see what it contained. It seems to be for a stomach upset.

'We need to stay in,' said John firmly. 'We are self-isolating. And because of my heart, I am shielding.' He has all the lingo off pat, and seems quite proud of it, but I think he gets mixed up sometimes.

Had soup for dinner, and drank orange juice – sort of comfort food.

More sad news about shops, pubs and restaurants going into administration, which will never open again. And some bosses of course are taking advantage of the furlough scheme to lay staff off. All that money some bosses took off us when times were good, and then they weren't there for us when times were bad. Rather like those who profited from the war.

Boris Johnson was moved into Intensive Care. Apparently we now have a national shortage of ventilators. Dyson are going to produce some. I hope they're better than the Dyson vacuum cleaner I had which blew up.

## Thursday April 9th

Couldn't be bothered to get up today. Stayed in bed and listened to the radio and read. I wasn't very hungry – ate mainly toast and soup. I was thirsty though. I thought a great deal about my symptoms. Catrin was never diagnosed as having CV. I am very prone to colds and coughs. I shouldn't think every time I feel unwell that I have Covid. Liz is terrible for this;

she apparently thinks it can creep in through the keyhole. I'm sure I will feel better tomorrow. Felt mildly sick.

*It was a very ill time to be sick in, for if any one complained, it was immediately said he had the plague ...* (Defoe)

## Friday April 10th

Good Friday, and the deli included hot cross buns in our home delivery. I did eat one with lots of butter on, so I'm hoping I've turned the corner. Still very thirsty and drank lots of orange juice ... And was immediately sick – just as Catrin was. So it is the same bug, whatever that is.

The death toll is rising. Some say it is higher than it is, as deaths in care homes are not being recorded as Covid-related.

## Saturday April 11th

I'd bought John and Catrin some chocolate from the Fairtrade shop before everything closed down, so John popped round with Catrin's and left it on the step.

Because of her heart, she is now 'shielding', thank goodness. GP advice.

A food bank is now running in the town.

Can no longer get to the bathroom, so John resignedly re-deployed the bowls and buckets he had used with Catrin.

## Sunday April 12th

Easter Sunday. Did not feel hungry at all, though John fetched me some grapes, and then ended up eating most of them himself. I was sick after I drank some milk. I have gone off tea and coffee completely. No church services. No church bells to ring out in celebration. Mom said they rang out to celebrate the end of the war. I do not know that they can ever ring out to celebrate the end of Coronavirus. The plague raged for hundreds of years.

The Spanish flu epidemic of 1919 raged for two years. They never found a vaccine for it; it simply ran its course. It killed more people than had died in World War I.

## Monday April 13th

Not hungry at all. Just tried to drink a lot. Terribly thirsty.

Heroic stories of family separation on the news – those who do essential work, for example for the National

Grid, and are living in pods away from their families. I thought about Defoe's conversation with a waterman, working to support the family he was separated from.

> *'But,' said I, 'why do you not come at them? How can you abandon your own flesh and blood?' 'Oh, sir,' says he, 'the Lord forbid! I do not abandon them; I work for them as much as I am able … I am a waterman, and there's my boat,' says he, 'and the boat serves me for a house. I work in it in the day, and I sleep in it in the night; and what I get I lay down upon that stone,' says he, showing me a broad stone on the other side of the street, a good way from his house; 'and then,' says he, 'I halloo, and call to them till I make them hear; and they come and fetch it.'* (Defoe)

## Tuesday April 14th

Tried to eat some toast for breakfast and was horribly sick straight after.

Same with soup at lunchtime. Had no dinner. Stayed in bed. John had to put a bucket next to it.

Boris Johnson has left hospital.

All our deliveries from the High Street shops in Abergele now left on the doorstep. They ring the bell and don't come near.

34

*... this necessity of going out of our houses to buy provisions was in a great measure the ruin of the whole city, for the people caught the distemper on these occasions one of another, and even the provisions themselves were often tainted ... (Defoe)*

## Wednesday April 15th

Wondering if I'll be well enough to go back to virtual work on Monday. The few things I tried to eat came up. Burning thirst, but didn't want any tea – drank juice.

Rumours that despite travel restrictions, lockdown and the prohibition of the use of holiday homes, some prominent people may indeed have left London. The Queen has gone to Windsor.

## Thursday April 16th

Slept very badly as I feel so odd – couldn't stand the feel of the quilt.

More stories of people breaking the lockdown. There are gatherings round here, in gardens and parks.

## Friday April 17th

Spent the whole day being sick. Asked John to get me

some Lucozade. The only time I like it is when I am unwell.

I don't think I have CV as I don't have any breathing problems, and I don't have a temperature. John is scanning NHS 100 anxiously for symptoms, but it doesn't mention sickness.

Haven't had the radio on for days, as I can't stand the noise anymore.

## Saturday April 18th

Slept badly, kept waking up with a burning thirst. Drank Lucozade, and brought it all up. Couldn't get to the loo as I am too weak to walk.

People around the world abandoned on cruise ships, which are apparently floating coffins.

## Sunday April 19th

On nothing but water now.

I took a few sips this morning, so I would not dehydrate. I've forgotten all about food – have not eaten for about 10 days now.

Ten minutes later, the water came up. I tried again, with the same result.

I stared at the bucket, and called for John.

As he came in, I said:

'It's time to go.'

He stared at me.

'What do you mean?'

'I need you to call for an ambulance.'

I didn't know I had made the decision until I said the words. I could have asked him to call the out-of-hours service. I could have asked him to take me to Accident and Emergency.

'Shall I call the GP?'

'It's Sunday. You know what happens. They refer it to an out-of-hours service, and they ask you to rate yourself on a one to ten.'

I suddenly realised why I needed an ambulance.

'I haven't eaten anything for ten days. I can't even hold water down now. And you can't take me because I can't get up. I can't get dressed. I can't go down the stairs, and I can't sit in the car.'

As he turned to go out the door, I added:

'And phone on your mobile. If they want to speak to me, I can't walk. I can't get to the phone.'

Not long after, I heard him on his mobile. I couldn't hear what he was saying, but then he came in.

'It's a nurse... she wants to speak to you.'

I hoped she was not going to ask me to rate myself on a one to ten. But she proved surprisingly sympathetic. Then she asked to speak to John again and he went out.

He came back, looking worried. I think that's when he really took my illness seriously for the first time. He'd thought, as you always do, that I would get better.

'She does think you need to be in hospital, and she's called an ambulance,' he said, looking stunned. I felt sorry for him.

'Get me ready to go... I can't get dressed. Bring me a dressing gown and slippers, and my little toiletries bag from the bathroom, and put a hairbrush into my bag.'

I don't know what last vestiges of vanity I had, that I got John to bring me a clean nightdress, and a new dressing gown, and the slippers that I always wear at Christmas.

This only took about twenty minutes, and then we heard the doorbell ring. I was surprised they were so quick, as you hear so many horror stories.

'I'm Owen, he's Glen,' one of two big men dressed in blue introduced themselves. 'We call ourselves Owen Glendower.' They both laughed. Both of them were wearing masks and gloves with their ordinary ambulance uniform. They didn't have aprons though.

I felt a bit embarrassed about being in my nightie. And the state of the bedroom. But I couldn't lift my head from the pillow.

They were very thorough. John explained about the sickness. They took my temperature and blood pressure, and conferred a bit. Then Glen said:

'You don't have much of a temperature and your blood pressure is pretty normal. But you can't eat or drink, and we think you're dehydrated. We think it's better if you go to hospital for observation.'

John looked ready to sink through the floor. I don't think he thought it would happen till it did.

Then there was the problem of getting me into the ambulance. I couldn't walk at all. Owen Glendower lifted me into a wheelchair and I was promptly sick. They didn't seem to mind. Owen gave me a bag to be sick into.

Then there was the problem of getting the chair down the stairs. They fetched some kind of small ramp from the ambulance and got me down a few steps at a time. Then they lifted the chair down the front steps, to where the ambulance was waiting. I could see the neighbours looking out of their windows.

Once I was inside the ambulance, they lifted me from the chair onto a bed, and strapped me down. Owen sat with me.

I could hear Glen talking to John.

'We can't take you in the ambulance. Visiting times are only fifteen minutes now, but you'll have to ring to see where she is.'

I struggled to raise my head as the doors were shut. I wanted to see the house and the outside world for the last time. I saw John's distraught face.

It was a short journey down the A55 to hospital. I clutched my sick bag.

'I've never been in an ambulance before,' I said to Owen. And had I not felt so ill, I would have liked to look around.

'We're taking you to A&E,' he said. 'So we'll be going round the back. Three quarters of the hospital is CV now, the rest is cancer, maternity and A&E.'

When we got there, we had to wait outside a locked door at the back for a while. Then Owen and Glen put me back into the chair, then onto a waiting trolley, and then lifted me into a bed in a small cubicle.

'You'll be fine now!'

I was sorry to see them go. I thought I might never see them again, and I hadn't thanked them enough.

Nobody took any notice of me for a bit. I could see other occupied beds, and staff moving around in gowns and masks. I felt quite peaceful. I didn't feel as tense as I did at home, where I felt I had to get well as soon as possible. I felt I was somewhere where I would be looked after.

Eventually, things started happening; I had my blood pressure checked and temperature taken, and various other pokes and prods. Then a young doctor came over to me. They all seemed so young.

'We'll keep you in for forty-eight hours, and give you anti-sickness medication,' he said.

As he finished, a male nurse joined him. He asked me to open my mouth; I did, and he inserted something into it.

'A swab,' he explained.

I was lifted onto a trolley again, and wheeled off through the hospital. We went through a huge set of double doors, which read:

## Ward Nine
## CORONAVIRUS
## No Unauthorised Entry

It did not say 'abandon all hope, ye who enter here.'

'We're just putting you in a side room here, as we're so short of beds,' explained one of the orderlies. 'We've got hardly any beds that aren't for CV.'

I'm glad they don't seem to think I have Covid. I still have hope – that I don't have the regular symptoms of Covid. That I have a stomach disorder. That I'll soon be home.

# PART TWO

## Monday April 20<sup>th</sup>

Ward Nine is apparently over its capacity, and one of the many wards in the hospital which now contains Coronavirus. But I'm in a small room with four other women, and this is not a Covid room.

When we got here, I was lifted into a hospital bed. They are very different to how I remember them. Mine has controls so you can raise and lower the head, and a control to call the nurse. Trouble is I don't want to raise my head. I think I have become worse since I came in.

I refused breakfast, which was brought in by a genial man called Tom. He went to every bed, and asked people what they wanted. Tom wears full PPE, but seems to be smiling through his mask. I took only an orange juice, as the burning thirst has returned. As soon as I drank it, through a straw, it came up.

Soon after, a nice blonde nurse came over to me. She was wearing a mask and gloves and a visor which looked like ski goggles (and perhaps was). Her long blue apron fell almost to the floor.

'I'm Susan,' she said. 'We're going to put you on a drip, and also anti-sickness medication.'

This involved having tubes fitted in my arms on both sides. I winced when the needles went in.

Another lady came to my bedside. She too was wearing an apron and a mask, and a scarf over her head, and gloves.

'I'm Maria,' she introduced herself. 'I'm your healthcare assistant. I'm going to help you with a wash.'

After drawing the curtains, she brought a bowl, towel and soap, and patiently washed my hands and face and arms. I didn't feel well enough to sit up, so she couldn't wash my body.

'I need to go to the toilet,' I whispered.

I don't know why; I'm not drinking. I suppose it is the drip.

'I will bring you a bedpan,' she said.

The bedpan turned out to be made of cardboard and she slid it into the bed. It's like being a child again.

I thanked her for all her care of me, and as she had a slight accent, I asked:

'Where do you come from originally?'

She smiled.

'Many people ask me that. I am from Belarus. But here, in this hospital, we are not from anywhere. We are a united army fighting Coronavirus. That is who we are.'

Turns out Maria has a degree in Russian literature, and is very philosophical. She is married to a Welshman. Working as a healthcare assistant is the only job she could get in the UK, but she told me she enjoys the practical aspects, which she dishes out with wise sayings.

At half past eight, Susan and the other nurse, Yasmin, left and the night shift arrived.

## Tuesday April 21st

Slept very badly. There is a lady, Dorothy, opposite me who has dementia. She snored very loudly. Machines kept going on and off.

The ward starts moving at six o'clock when the night shift come around and start taking our blood pressure and temperature before they clock off.

Tom came to offer breakfast, and I refused everything

except a little orange juice in a carton. He looked a bit concerned. But I am not hungry at all.

Lay flat on my back, feeling sick.

Susan and Yasmin arrived at eight thirty. I watched them put on their masks, gowns and gloves. Yasmin also has a scarf tied around her hair.

'The doctors are coming round today,' she told me.

The ward was cleaned by a young man. Pushing around a huge broom, he told me his name was Jan, and he was from Poland.

'This is the only job I can get, but I am proud to do it,' he said.

When the doctor arrived, he pulled the curtains around the bed. He had a few young people with him, and I supposed they were medical students. He introduced himself as Dr Mohammed. But he seemed very young as well.

'I am sorry to tell you that your test was positive,' he said gently. 'You have Coronavirus. We shall be keeping you in for a short time.'

After they went, I lay in bed thinking about it. I had never thought it was Coronavirus... or had I? I told myself Catrin had a cold, or gastroenteritis. I blocked it from my mind. I just didn't want to know the truth. I fooled myself. And you never think it will happen to you. It seemed odd to think you had something that might kill you.

I felt a goose walk, very softly, over my grave. I looked at the window, expecting the Four Horsemen of the Apocalypse to ride by. War. Famine. Disease. Death.

All that time when nothing seemed to be happening. It was like the Phony War, as Mom always said, and you were lulled into a sense of false security. And then it was the Blitz, and everything was happening at once. Death and destruction.

*And here I must observe also that the plague, as I suppose all distempers do, operated in a different manner on differing constitutions; some were immediately overwhelmed with it, and it came to violent fevers, vomitings, insufferable headaches, pains in the back, and so up to ravings and ragings … while others, as I have observed, were silently infected, the fever preying upon their spirits insensibly…* (Defoe)

I could see my bag on the table next to the bed. It is all I have, along with my nightdress and dressing gown and slippers. I have nothing else.

Susan told me gently that nobody on the ward could have visitors. I am surrounded by staff and patients I

47

don't know... it feels oddly like the first day at a new school, but far worse. I have never felt quite so alone in my life.

Two of the patients in my room were put onto trolleys and taken out, and then two more women wheeled in.

'This is now a Coronavirus ward,' said Susan.

*Every visited House to be marked.*
*'That every house visited be marked with a red cross of a foot long in the middle of the door ...'*
(Defoe)

She fitted a large oxygen mask over my face. She said it will help me to breathe, that my saturation level needs to be higher. Or 'sats' as she called it, and I had to ask what that was. It is another of the new terms I have learned. Now I have holes in each arm and a mask strapped to my face.

I'm not really struggling to breathe as some of the other women are. Of course, wherever you go, it goes with you – I've watched them being pushed in wheelchairs to the bathroom with their equipment solemnly accompanying them.

The silver cylinders which come with us when we move say British Oxygen Cylinder. This was an observation which I found very comforting. It reminded me that Dad had worked for the BOC in his youth, fitting oxygen equipment into hospitals. Whenever we drove past a hospital, he'd wave proudly: 'I put the oxygen equipment in there!'

Susan told me that John and Liz had phoned the hospital. I hadn't thought of them at all. I feel too unwell to talk to anyone – or reassure them that I am getting better.

Refused lunch and dinner.

Lay alone in the dark, surrounded by people.

## Wednesday April 22nd

Had a bad night as the tubes in my arms hurt so much. I cried a bit, and buzzed for one of the night nurses, who came quickly. They turn the lights down at night, and like everyone else, the nurses have their faces and head covered – so you never see their faces and don't know who they are. If they are wearing badges, it's too dark to see them. You can only see their eyes, gleaming in the blackness. The night nurse gave me some liquid paracetamol in a tiny cup.

I had to ask also to use the bedpan in the night. I hate having to trouble them about this. The worst is if you spill, and they have to change all of the bedclothes. They never make a fuss.

Refused breakfast, apart from orange juice. I only have this because of my terrible burning thirst. But I can only take one tiny sip at a time, in an effort not to be sick.

Two new nurses arrived today: Natalie, who is very young, and a middle-aged lady called Izabella, who told me she is Romanian. She said the nurses do three days on, three days off, eight thirty till eight thirty, half hour for lunch and – if they're lucky – fifteen minutes in the morning and afternoon for a tea break. Natalie has the bloom of youth, and the bounce. She is Life. She is Immortal. She told me she was a nurse in a clinic, but has now volunteered to work in the hospital due to staff shortages.

'The staff cafe is closed, so we have to bring our own food in, and catering will bring us a cup of tea if we phone down,' said Izabella.

I think the staff in this hospital come from all over the world. If the 'Send them Back' Brigade had their way, the hospital could hardly operate.

My nightdress is dirty now. Izabella pulled the curtains, and managed to get it off. She gave me a gown to wear. It is marked For Hospital Use only, and is open at the back, with a couple of ties.

Natalie gave me something called a Nutrisip, a strawberry drink in a plastic bottle with a straw. I sipped it – and it was quite nice, like a milk shake. Then it came straight up, into my cardboard bowl.

Natalie sighed as she replaced the bowl.

'Your condition is *abysmal*,' she said.

Izabella reported that John and Liz had both called. I have switched my phone off because I don't feel well enough to talk to them. I don't want to talk to them. I have nothing to say that isn't depressing. I don't have the energy. I can only cope with the people who now look after me. And it's as though it's another world, outside. I live in the hospital now. I am a sick person. My world is nothing but my hospital bed. And a little room in Ward Nine: Coronavirus. Which is full of strangers.

I felt guilty for not getting better. I've had needles in each arm, anti-sickness medication and a drip. I have an oxygen mask. I have liquid paracetamol in a tiny cup, and every so often, I have an injection in my tummy. I have a funny taste in my mouth, a runny nose, and I feel muggy, as though I have the flu. I have constant and debilitating sickness. But I don't have treatment for Coronavirus because there is none.

Refused dinner. Dorothy, the lady with dementia, snored so badly in the night that myself and the lady opposite, Jane, had to call the nurse and ask for her to be removed.

I had introduced myself to Jane when she shuffled over to use the bathroom. I sort of feel I need friends on the ward, that we should all have something in common (which we have — Coronavirus). We are thrown together by circumstance and sickness. Efforts at conversation are polite and quite stressful.

The night shift had to come and load Dorothy onto a trolley. We felt bad about doing that, but as Jane said, we couldn't get any sleep at all.

Dorothy's family used to phone her on her mobile, and the nurses would hold it up for her. They would put it on speaker, and you could hear the family telling her they loved her. But I don't think she even knew who they were.

## Thursday April 23rd

Terrible choking episode today. Ate nothing. Wanted to die.

It happened after lunch. I went to sleep – I hardly sleep at night, as there is so much going on. So my sleeping patterns have changed entirely.

I had been drifting, somewhere, towards something, when I came back to consciousness with a start. There was a light, but it was the glaring overhead light of Ward Nine. I was in my hospital bed, and being held up and forward. Somebody – a man in full PPE – was kneeling behind me on the bed. There were sharp blows on my back, and his fists were closed in front of me.

I was choking, and then it all came up, into the basin that Nurse Susan was holding in front of me.

Later, when the nurses had changed my gown and all the bedsheets, she came over to me.

'You stopped breathing,' she said. 'We called for the doctor, and when he came, he said you were choking on your own vomit in your sleep.'

Susan came closer.

'You need to *try*,' she said gently. 'You need to *try* so you can get better. Please *try* for me. And all of us.'

I closed my eyes.

'Sue,' I said at last, 'I honestly don't care anymore. If I could close my eyes and just drift away, I would. I think I actually want to die. I can't stand it any longer.'

I opened my eyes. She was staring at me, and I think there were tears in her eyes. She knows I have almost given up and they are doing everything they can.

Later on, Dr Mohammed and some others stood at the end of my bed. I could hear them whispering.

'The Intensive Care Unit ...'

Most people who come to this ward come from the ICU. I may be the first person who goes from here to ICU. My symptoms are previously unknown.

> *I am not physician enough to enter into the partic-*
> *ular reasons and manner of these differing effects*
> *of one and the same distemper, and of its differing*
> *operation in several bodies; nor is it my business*
> *here to record the observations which I really made,*
> *because the doctors themselves have done that part*
> *much more effectually than I can do ...* (Defoe)

## Friday April 24th

Two nurses arrived at my bed with a very large piece of equipment with some clear tubes coming out of it.

Natalie came up to the bed.

'We want to try and feed you nasogastrically,' she explained. 'We fit the tubes via your nose, and they go into your stomach.'

I didn't like the sound of that at all.

'I think I'd rather not,' I said.

'Look,' said Natalie impatiently, 'your condition is

*abysmal*, I've said that before. We have to do this.' I think abysmal is her favourite word.

After some arguing, and a few tears, I consented.

The tubes were inserted into my nose. After only a few seconds I could hear a voice screaming, 'No, no, no!' I realised it was me.

I pulled the tubes out.

I opened my eyes. The two nurses looked shocked, and both Natalie and Izabella were hovering anxiously.

Izabella held my hand.

'We really have to try ... after the choking yesterday ...'

The second time was even worse, and now as I screamed, I disturbed the room, probably the whole ward, and the nurses went away.

'Look,' one of them said before she went. 'We have somebody in on Monday who's really expert on doing this, and we can sedate you too.'

It sounded like a threat.

I felt I had reached rock bottom. I lay in bed with tears in my eyes. I felt I had caused trouble, that they were only trying to help.

I heard Natalie on the phone to John. The phone is only on the other side of the room. He must have phoned to see how I am; I'm still not up to phoning anyone. I could only hear Natalie.

'Thank you for calling. No, it's not good. Yes, I'm sorry. She can't eat anything at all. The drip isn't enough anymore. We tried artificial feeding, and she pulled it out. We're going to need your permission to continue. Otherwise, it could be very bad. And we think she might need to go now to the Intensive Care Unit. What worries us is that she's not *trying* ...'
Natalie sounded hopeless.

I made up my mind. I must start to eat. I must help the staff.

## Saturday April 25th

Tom came in with the breakfast and looked at me helplessly.

'Anything for breakfast? We have cereal, we have porridge, we have yoghurts, we have toast.'

'I think I'll try a yoghurt today, and an orange juice,' I said.

He stared at me. I can't see much of his face, or anybody's face because they all wear masks. But I could see from the way his eyes crinkled up that he had broken into a huge smile.

I realised that he really cared whether I ate or not.

The yoghurt was lovely, though I have a funny taste in my mouth, and Tom gave me two orange juices because of my terrible thirst.

I lay back, holding my cardboard bowl, and waited to be sick.

And I wasn't.

I couldn't believe it at first. I lay there, expecting it any moment. It has always been immediate, and about mid-morning, I began to hope.

I lay looking out of the window – we have a view of hills, luckily. *I will look up to the hills, from whence comes my help.* We had that at school. Does the help come from the hills though, or is it a statement of despair – a question?

Tom came again at lunchtime, looking optimistic. I didn't feel quite ready for the hot food, but to please him, I did take another yoghurt, and a little cheesecake, which I actually enjoyed.

Yasmin came bouncing over, beaming.

'This is really good! I want you to have some Nutrisips – you can have strawberry, chocolate and banana, and they'll be really good for you!'

They come in a little plastic bottle with a straw. I chose strawberry.

Slept all afternoon, which you do when you are awake in the night. Then, I actually woke up feeling hungry. Tom offered me a jacket potato, which I really enjoyed. He was beaming again when he came for the rubbish. He really cares.

Lights out at nine o'clock. I had to buzz for the nurse a couple of times in the night as I needed the bathroom. It's a relief not to use the bedpan, but my oxygen cylinder has to go where I go.

## Sunday April 26th

It is very quiet at the weekends, as the doctors don't come round. I lay in bed, looking out of the window.

I wondered if there was a chapel in the hospital, as there used to be. My physiotherapy appointments for arthritis are at Rhyl, and once when I was walking along the corridor I saw a door labelled Chapel. I looked inside and it was beautiful – all polished wood and stained glass. There was even an organ, with a pile of leaflets for a Carol Service in 1996 on it – probably the last time it was used for a service, as the hospital is no longer a bedded one. After that, I always used to sit quietly in there for a bit whenever I went for physio.

Looking around, I noticed a small plastic pocket on the table next my bed. There was a book in it. I pulled it out and it was a Gideon Bible. I remember the fuss when they stopped putting them out in rooms in Travelodge. I don't think anyone here has noticed it. No ministers can visit the sick here.

> *Some of the ministers did visit the sick at first and for a little while, but it was not to be done. It would have been present death to have gone into some houses.* (Defoe)

Sunday breakfast was brought by a nice young man called Qasim. He was from Syria, he said, and had come here fleeing the war. He loved his NHS job.

I said I would be proud to do any job at all for them.

At Qasim's urging, I progressed beyond a breakfast yoghurt and orange juice, and tried some toast and tea. The tea tasted awful, which might be my mouth, but I haven't had tea in nearly two weeks. Qasim was beaming when he came up for the rubbish. It struck me that the catering staff act almost as dieticians. I suppose they are what the Government call low-skilled workers.

Word had obviously been around, as Maria, my healthcare assistant, also came up beaming.

'No bed bath today! We will take you to the bathroom!'

'Oh Maria, I don't fancy that at all.'

She looked disappointed, and I felt suddenly guilty. Why does their good opinion mean so much? Because they care. Because I'm not trying. Because they're the grown-ups and I'm the child. I am so used to looking after people, being the mother figure, the one who is the carer – even to my Mom when she was old and ill. And now I am being cared for.

Maria fetched me a wheelchair. I sat on the edge of the bed, and leaned forward to get into it. I felt very weak. And as I moved, I was suddenly sick.

Maria was distressed, I could see. She wears a transparent ski mask, so you can see her face.

'Don't worry, I will get you a clean gown. It was too much!'

She drew the curtains. Yasmin and Susan came and changed all my bedclothes, and never said a word about it. Maria came back beaming, with an armful of nightwear, all colours, and brand new.

'Look! This will cheer you up! We have a donation from Marks and Spencer!'

Turns out M&S have donated dressing gowns, nighties and pyjamas to the hospital; I suppose they can't sell it. I had a blue nightie and dressing gown, and they're nicer than anything I have ever had. You have so little in hospital that everything means something. I have a nightie and dressing gown in a plastic bag marked Patient Property, a pair of slippers and a handbag with a purse, hairbrush and phone inside. I have nothing else. I am stripped to the bare essentials.

After the sickness, I lay quietly till lunch time. Maria brought me a cup of tea, which was horrible, and some ginger biscuits in a little packet.

'Donated by a local supermarket,' she explained. I thought how kind some people were.

Thanks to Qasim's encouragement, managed to eat cheese sandwiches for lunch and soup for tea. Yasmin made a face when she saw it.

'I'm sorry for the food,' she said bluntly.

'Oh Yasmin, I quite like it, after not eating for so long. And to be honest, I'm just relieved I don't have to pay for it! I'll go out of here without owing anyone a penny!'

I do like it – there is curry and pasta on offer, but I also like the traditional foods which remind me in a comforting way of Mom's cooking in the 1960s (which was very good) and school dinners in the 1970s (not so good). Tom and Qasim stand at the door, as the trolley is left outside. They announce the menu to the room, which gives you time to think what you want, and the announcement either cheers us up or plunges us into the depths of despair, depending what's on offer. The healthcare assistants should then bring the food to our bed tables, but they are so busy on the ward that Tom and Qasim often help out with this. Just as the nurses and healthcare assistants help each other out. They are working at full stretch.

Reports on the news of people breaking lockdown. Raves, barbeques, secret visits to second homes.

*What variety of stratagems were used to escape and get out of houses thus shut up, by which the watchmen were deceived or overpowered, and that the people got away, I have taken notice of already, and shall say no more to that.* (Defoe)

## Monday April 27th

Now that I am feeling a bit better, I have started to notice how the daily routine of the ward carries on, as usual, in the face of life and death.

I have gotten used to not sleeping at night. They lower the lights at nine o'clock, but there is always something going on in the ward, always machines bleeping, always nurses coming round.

We start at six o'clock, with our temperatures taken and blood pressure checked. Some people don't like that – the feel of something tightening round your arm – but I don't mind it. They use your ear to take your temperature now.

Big day today! Dr Mohammed made his rounds and said I could have the drip and the anti-sickness medication removed! Dr Mohammed is always accompanied by an admiring coterie of students who have graduated early to join the frontline.

Yasmin and Sue took the tubes out. I have had so many needles inserted in my arms that they are a mass of tiny scars. But it was wonderful to be able to move my arms again, even if they are sore.

Susan also took away the big oxygen mask, and gave me a cylinder with two plastic tubes attached, which I had to put up my nose. I actually found this more uncomfortable than the big mask.

'Your sats are still a bit low,' she explained.

The tubes reminded me of how only a few days ago, they were trying to insert tubes into my nose and into

my stomach, and how I kicked and screamed. I
realised humbly that I would not have been able to be
a suffragette undergoing force feeding. It was the
turning point in many ways – I forced myself to eat to
avoid the tubes. Now everyone is very pleased with
me. It is like being a good child at school, and very
comforting in a way. Because I don't know what I need
to do to recover from CV.

Tom back, and found out that I actually now look
forward to meal times. It's odd how it is served – in
cardboard containers, and with plastic cutlery. I don't
know if this is because of CV, or if it's the norm now.
Years ago, when I was a student, I had a holiday job in
a hospital and part of my job was loading huge
dishwashers with crockery and cutlery.

Maria was off today, and I had a healthcare assistant
called Fatima. She is very brisk.

'We are going to the bathroom today,' she announced
firmly via her ski mask.

She brought a wheelchair to the bedside and helped me
into it. This time I wasn't sick. She wheeled me to the
bathroom, which is just at the end of our side room,
which is one of many on the ward. It is a large and
very light room, with a loo and an overhead shower.

'You can just sit under the shower, and I'll wash your
hair,' Fatima urged.

But I didn't feel ready for that, although my hair is indeed dreadful. So I just had a wash at the sink. Fatima brought me a new toothbrush, because it was one of the things I forgot to bring in with me. I felt quite pleased to have a brand new yellow toothbrush. I arranged it carefully on the little table next to my bed, which Fatima drew up closer to the bed for me.

Izabella came up after lunch.

'Now your husband and sister phone every day, and always we tell them how you are, but it takes time to answer the phone. So I think today we tell them to phone you on your mobile,' she said firmly.

'It's in my bag, Izabella, and must be as flat as a pancake.'

Izabella found it for me, and plugged it in at my table, where it is next to all sorts of important-looking plugs. I hope I don't pull the wrong plug out by mistake.

Izabella also suggested that I sit in my chair for a bit. I didn't fancy this. I like to just lie on my bed and look out the window. But Izabella insisted.

'You can breathe better sitting up,' she said firmly.

So she helped me into the chair, and put a pillow behind me. Then she brushed my hair, which was a terrible mess, and has grown so much that she went and found a ribbon to tie it back for me.

'Much better!' she beamed.

I have nothing to read, but I don't want to. I don't have the mental application. I would never have thought that. I remember years ago when I worked for the public library service, we used to loan books to hospitals in partnership with the RVS[1]. And when Mom and Dad were in, a trolley used to come around with newspapers and magazines. But we are isolated.

I tried not to look at the three other women on the ward. The lady opposite, Mary, seems in a bad way, asleep all the time. Jane, who came in from Intensive Care, is now quite lively, and smiled and waved. She hopes to go home soon. Jenny next to me suffers from depression, and sits and looks at the floor all the time. She never smiles. I remember when I used to visit Mom in hospital, I used to think how all the old ladies looked sad and depressed, and I wondered why. But now I think I know.

It is hard to get to know anyone, though. They come and go all the time, on their way home, to other wards, to the ICU, or to the mortuary.

At lunchtime, Tom tried to wake Mary and feed her patiently spoon by spoon, as the healthcare assistants were run off their feet. It was obviously hopeless, and they drew her curtains and brought a drip.

---

[1] Royal Voluntary Service formerly Women's Royal Voluntary Service

My phone rang twice in the afternoon. It was John and then Liz. It was odd to speak to them. I don't know if I was pleased or not. It's as though they came from another world. I couldn't tell them the things that had happened to me. They wouldn't understand.

Liz was emotional.

'We've been so worried... I've been trying your phone so long... I phoned the ward *every* day... I kept thinking, you're my only sister, and the only one left who remembers the old days... Graham and the lads send all their love... I thought the worst. Every time the phone rang, I thought this is it...'

She ended up in tears, as did I. You see, I was the elder sister. I was not supposed to be ill... Mom would send us out to play, saying: 'Look after your little sister.'

John tried hard not to be emotional. Stiff upper lip.

'I've phoned the ward every day. They said you had stopped *trying*.' He cleared his throat and stopped for a minute, then went on gamely. 'The cats are all well. I keep in touch with Catrin.' He stopped.

'I wish you would come home.'

Much hilarity on the ward today, as Donald Trump has suggested injecting bleach as a cure for Coronavirus, and even Dr Mohammed was unable to hide his smiles.

*... they ran to conjurers and witches, and all sorts of deceivers, to know what should become of them (who fed their fears, and kept them always alarmed and awake on purpose to delude them and pick their pockets) ... storing themselves with such multitudes of pills, potions, and preservatives, as they were called, that they not only spent their money but even poisoned themselves beforehand for fear of the poison of the infection ...* (Defoe)

## Tuesday April 28th

Something odd happened in the night.

Lights go out at nine o'clock, and now all the tubes have been removed from my arms, I can actually doze off. I have to lie flat on my back because of the tubes in my nose.

About three o'clock, I woke up to the sound of a machine bleeping very fast. The room was full of people in gowns and masks, and they drew the curtains around Mary's bed. Then, after some time, they all went away and there was silence. Then one of the night nurses came and pulled back the curtains.

Two men arrived with a trolley. They lifted Mary onto it. The night nurse covered her with a white sheet. Then they wheeled her away.

The night nurse turned around and saw me staring.

'We don't even have enough body bags,' she said.

Her eyes seemed bright; I think she was crying. To me, in that dark hospital room, she seemed like the Angel of Death.

Nobody mentioned Mary in the morning; not the other women, who stared at the empty bed, nor the day staff. I was especially conscientious about wearing my breathing equipment. I think I realised for the first time that whatever the staff tried to do, they could not necessarily save you. Death stalks the ward. Here, we are as close to the dead as the living.

> *Doubtless, the physicians assisted many by their skill, and by their prudence and applications, to the saving of their lives and restoring their health. But it is not lessening their character or their skill, to say they could not cure those that had the tokens upon them, or those who were mortally infected before the physicians were sent for, as was frequently the case.* (Defoe)

## Wednesday April 29th

A nice young woman called Kay came to see me today. She introduced herself as a dietician. She gave me a diet booklet, which is rather lovely; it is full of things like milk shakes and cakes. I showed it to Tom, and he laughed and said he'd make sure I got everything in it. Fattening me for the kill, I suppose – or for leaving hospital.

Leaving hospital.

'You need to put weight back on,' she explained. This is the first time anybody has said this to me since I was a skinny child, suffering from catarrh and bronchitis, in a damp terraced house. The health visitor had told my mom I needed cod liver oil and Delrosa. I remember Liz and I had to drink pasteurised milk and orange juice every day; we didn't care for it at all.

In the afternoon I dozed off and woke rather abruptly to find two people standing at my bedside. They wore white rather than blue. One was a young and cheerful man called Matt, and the other a middle-aged lady called Bev.

'We're Physiotherapy. We're here to help you get back on your feet!'

My heart sank at this. I only move, with help, from my bed to my chair, and into my wheelchair. I can now be wheeled to the bathroom, which is good because the bedpan was a total flop and I could never use it without an accident.

'I don't think I can walk...' I told them. 'I am so weak.'

'Of course you are, your muscles are wasted,' said Matt cheerfully.

He produced, almost with a flourish, a Zimmer frame, which they had left at the entrance to the ward. I looked at it aghast.

'A Zimmer! That's for old women!'

They laughed, and in that dreadful moment, I realised I was an old woman.

'Just a few steps... just try a little walk... just to the bathroom and back...'

I realised I was behaving like a spoilt child, and they were behaving like the grown-ups. And so to please them, and to get some peace, I levered myself up and made some faltering steps down the ward. I did about six, and said:

'That's enough. I've had enough.'

They were very pleased though. They said they would be back tomorrow, and would bring me a stick. They left me some exercises to do, in bed and in my chair. I think I'll stick to the bed exercises.

I have heard that the mortuary here is quite full. 'Corpses stacked high,' said my informant ghoulishly. 'They're using shipping containers in the outside world.'

> *... seeing they were all dead, and were to be huddled together into the common grave of mankind, as we may call it, for here was no difference made, but poor and rich went together; there was no other way of burials, neither was it possible there should, for coffins were not to be had for the prodigious numbers that fell in such a calamity as this.* (Defoe)

## Thursday April 30th

Today's visitor was another very nice young woman called Claire, who said she was from Occupational Therapy. She asked me if there was anything I wanted to do, anything she could bring me.

'No,' I said.

She looked worried, and once again I felt that I wasn't trying hard enough. I cast around a bit and said that I liked reading, and listening to the radio. She seemed relieved at that.

'We can get you a radio!'

I was pleased, thinking that if they brought earphones,

I could lie or sit and listen to *Woman's Hour* and the afternoon play on Radio Four. What happened in fact was that Natalie brought in a huge radio, put it on the window, and the four of us listened in absolute indifference to a station called something like Kiss Kiss FM. Natalie seemed to like it though, and sang along to it, and the others seemed to like her singing. There is a lady called Edna, in a wheelchair, and Natalie did wheelchair dances with her and Edna laughed.

Claire did suggest that I wrote down some of my experiences, when I said I'd kept a diary in the past. She said it might prove therapeutic. And I said it might provide a record.

> *Such intervals as I had I employed in reading books and in writing down my memorandums of what occurred to me every day, and out of which afterwards I took most of this work, as it relates to my observations without doors.* (Defoe)

Afternoon brought Matt and Bev, accompanied by my stick, which is made of metal, not wood, and is adjustable. I used it to walk as far as the bathroom and back, and they were thrilled. I wasn't, but it will be great not to have to call the nurses for either the bedpan or the wheelchair. Baby steps. Learning to walk again.

'When you can walk the length of the ward, you can go home!' promised Bev.

Go home. Leave hospital.

Natalie turned the radio off when we had our afternoon naps, but obviously inspired by the success of Occupational Therapy's experiment in media, she turned the TV on after tea (lasagne and chips and chocolate mousses, announced to the ward by Tom with a flourish). This inspired a hunt all over the ward to find the remote control, and I can honestly say I wish she hadn't found it. The first thing that came on was the Government press conference, which was drivel. I have never seen so many people avoid so many questions in my life.

There was a succession of increasingly awful soap operas and reality programmes, but at 8pm, Natalie did put on The Clap for the NHS, which we watched in silence.

'I suppose you're really pleased at the appreciation,' I ventured to Natalie.

She shrugged her shoulders indifferently.

'Clapping costs nothing, and the politicians stand there and it makes them look good. Especially if the press turns up. What I'd like is a decent pay rise. And while they're at it, they could write off our student debt. I owe thousands in student loans.'

She began to peel off her gloves, ready for the

changeover. Her hands were red and raw, and I looked at them in horror. She laughed.

'That's what happens when you wear rubber gloves all day! And I wear two pairs! Still, I'm glad to have them, there's enough here haven't got the right equipment.'

I've thought for a long time how awful it is for them, in this heat, wearing masks, gloves and aprons that cover them from head to foot. And then I thought how some of the nurses wear ski masks instead of masks, and wrap scarves round their heads. And some have plastic aprons, almost like bin bags. And I thought how very few of them have PPE that goes from their necks to the floor, as they should do, but that the Westminster Government had downgraded what PPE was needed to fight Coronavirus. And what Maria had said about them being an army being sent into battle... They are an army without the right equipment.

Well, it's not the first time in this country that innocents have been sent over the top to be slaughtered.

## Friday May 1st

A new patient arrived today, a lady called Edith. She has dementia, and she has an alarm attached to her that goes off when she tries to get out of bed. She tried at first, and it went off constantly, and then she just gave up and lay back and closed her eyes. She seems in a bad way.

There was also a new nurse today, a Portuguese lady called Rosa, in her thirties, and very cheerful.

'Where's Izabella?' I asked Susan.

She looked around.

'She's in Intensive Care,' she whispered. 'She began to feel really ill at home and had to go to bed. She had terrible breathing problems. Her husband took her to A & E to get tested – it's not routine see – and she was positive.'

They must live with it all the time. Physician, heal thyself.

> *So the Plague defied all medicines; the very physicians were seized with it, with their preservatives in their mouths; and men went about prescribing to others and telling them what to do till the tokens were upon them, and they dropped down dead, destroyed by that very enemy they directed others to oppose.'* (Defoe)

Dr Mohammed came around with his students. He seems terribly impressed by my symptoms; he told me they'd never had a patient before whose main symptom was excessive vomiting. He wants to put

me into a paper he is writing for *The Lancet*, as
Patient A.

'We're making it up as we go along,' I heard him say to
the students as he strolled off.

Chatted a little bit with the lady next to me, Jean. She
hopes to go home soon. She told me she worked as a
carer in a care home.

'Most of us here, from the care homes. It's rampant,
and we get no testing,' she said bluntly. 'And they
don't always put CV on the death certificate. It's a
vicious circle; they get it, they come in here, we catch
it from them, and we end up in here. And then we go
back. Because if I don't work, I don't get paid. And I
am needed."

Jean is sixty-three. She told me she needs to work till
she is sixty-six and gets her state pension, as all they
have is her husband's state pension.

'I have a very small private pension,' I said doubtfully.

Jean laughed.

'I got married young, had the kids, looked after them
and my husband, did jobs that fitted in with their day
– cleaning, care, dinner lady. Never earned enough to
pay into a private pension. Then when I was older, I
had Mum and Dad to look after – I saved this country

thousands in care fees. Then they kicked me in the teeth and took my pension away that I'd worked and paid tax for. And us who do these jobs, we're in the line of fire. It could kill us.'

Jean had breathing problems at home, so bad that her husband took her to A&E, where she was sent straight to the ICU. She spent several days on a ventilator, and never knew a thing.

> *The women and servants that were turned off from their places were likewise employed as nurses to tend the sick in all places, and this took off a very great number of them.* (Defoe)

I thought about a young woman, Hayley, who came onto the ward yesterday. People come to A&E and say they might have the CV. They get a test and come onto the ward, and wait forty-eight hours for the result. If it's positive, and they're not too bad, they have the chance to stay or go home and self-isolate.

I'd seen Hayley getting dressed to go home, and I was surprised, as she didn't look too well at all. She saw me looking.

'I have to go,' she said tearfully. 'My husband's a long-distance delivery driver. If he don't work, he don't get paid. And he thinks he has to do what he does. And if I don't go home, he has to look after the kids, and he can't work. And now he can't come home for two weeks.'

The terrible choices people have to make. So many key workers, doing essential jobs, low pay or no pay. Nurses saddled with debt and risking their lives. Whose fault is that?

Visits from Kay, Claire and Matt and Bev, who were ecstatic when I wobbled halfway up the ward on my stick.

I told Claire the TV and radio experiments had been unsuccessful, and she gave me a book of word searches, produced by the hospital. We can't have books, she explained, because of the quarantine. But I don't want to read anyway. I can't concentrate. I feel sort of drained all the time.

Death toll rising steadily, but said to be even higher than they say it is.

## Saturday May 2nd

Was awoken in the night several times by Edith trying to get up and her alarm going off. The nurses would always come straight away.

Rosa and Susan were on today, and I heard them whispering.

'They always try and get up at the end...'

They saw me listening and stopped.

Yesterday, Edith's husband, son and daughter phoned several times, and the nurses put it on speaker, but she was incapable of having a conversation, and I could hear her daughter crying.

Today, Susan bought in an iPad.

'It's for a Zoom meeting,' she explained to me. 'It's so Edith's family can see her and say—' and she stopped.

During the daytime, either Rosa or Susan sat with Edith. She managed to wake up enough to look at the iPad – I'm not sure she understood what it was. But then, when her family came on, the most beautiful smile came over her face, and she chattered away.

It reminded me of when Dad was in the hospice. He was in a coma for the last two weeks, nothing there at all. One afternoon I sat very quietly with him, and when it was time to go, I bent over and kissed him and told him that I loved him. And at that moment, he opened his blue eyes wide and smiled at me. He knew me, just for a second. And then he was gone.

He died that night, and Liz and I went to the hospice to sit quietly with his body for a time.

At least we were able to visit. Nobody visits me. And nobody can visit Edith.

Qasim looked at her when he came in with the food. Qasim has tried to sit with her and feed her, patiently, spoon by spoon, when the HCAs were busy with others. Today, he shook his head and whispered something to Susan, and shortly afterwards she brought in a drip for Edith.

## Sunday May 3rd

Full turn-out of staff today. Yasmin, Natalie, Maria and Fatima. Usually, they are bustling around all the time and never sit down. I remembered what Susan had said when Boris Johnson made his sentimental speech about the two nurses who sat at his bedside.

'Luxury to have a nurse at your bedside twenty-four hours! We've got 120 to look after!'

But today the four were around most of the time. They took it in turns to sit next to Edith, holding her hand. She was mumbling, but a few words were coherent.

No professional visitors on Sunday, so Fatima took me to the bathroom and then helped me with my walking exercises. Using my stick, I got as far as the window. It was a beautiful day, and Qasim had opened the window to let in the fresh air. Leaning on Fatima, I looked out. Below, in the hospital grounds, a small group of people were standing under our window, looking up.

'It's Edith's family,' said Fatima bluntly.

They stood there all day. I don't know what they did for food and drink.

Edith was rambling now. She seemed to be talking to her mum and dad, and other long gone people. I remember, when I choked, hearing Mom's and Dad's voices. We are all children here.

And then some time in the afternoon, all her machines stopped making a noise.

There was total silence on the ward. We all looked. It was Fatima sitting there, holding her hand, and staring at her.

Yasmin went over and whispered something. She drew the curtains.

> *I could give several relations of good, pious, and religious people who, when they have had the distemper ... have forbid their own family to come near them, in hopes of their being preserved, and have even died without seeing their nearest relations lest they should be instrumental to give them the distemper, and infect or endanger them.* (Defoe)

Natalie was writing something on a large piece of paper. She took it over to the window, looked down, held it up, and stood there for some minutes. She raised her hand in salute.

When she turned round, I had a glimpse of what it said.

*SHE IS AT PEACE NOW. WE ARE ALL SO SORRY.*

## Monday May 4th

Very quiet on the ward today, after they took Edith away. I saw on the news that funerals are limited to six people. There were more than that outside her window.

> *Burial of the Dead.*
> *'... no neighbours nor friends be suffered to accompany the corpse to church, or to enter the house visited, upon pain of having his house shut up or be imprisoned... And further, all public assemblies at other burials are to be foreborne during the continuance of this visitation.'* (Defoe)

Women come and go all the time, and I've stopped trying to strike up relationships with them. We do have one thing in common – we are sick. But apart from that, conversation can be difficult, and so many of them are depressed, or have dementia. But the ward staff stay the same. Dr Mohammed, Natalie, Susan, Yasmin, Rosa, Izabella, Fatima, Maria, Tom, Qasim,

Jan, Matt, Beverley, Claire, Kay. They are my family now. I feel safe with them.

Dr Mohammed made his rounds. He looked at Edith's empty bed but said nothing. There will always be another patient for them. He looked at my notes and asked me how I'd enjoyed the experiment with Occupational Therapy and radio. I said Radio Kiss Kiss FM had been appalling, and he laughed and said he was a Radio Two and Five Live man himself. He particularly misses the football, and is a Man City fan.

He said wistfully:

'What I miss most is Sky Sports on a Saturday afternoon. I'd give anything to be sat there on the sofa again watching Paul Merson and the lads. I just put it on in the hope that something – anything – might be on, like the 1970 Cup Final. And then last week, it was Dion Dublin reminiscing about his times on *Homes under the Hammer*.' He shook his head sadly.

He said that I could have the breathing equipment removed, that my sats were normal.

'You can think about going home now!' he said.

Perhaps, after Edith's death, it is time to go home. But am I cured? Am I immune? Why did I get it? And will I get it again?

*I often reflected upon the unprovided condition that the whole body of the people were in at the first coming of this calamity upon them ... such a prodigious number of people sank in that disaster, which, if proper steps had been taken, might, Providence concurring, have been avoided, and which ... they may take a caution and warning from.* (Defoe)

Dr Mohammed, still murmuring something about Sky Sports, drifted off mournfully, followed at a respectful distance by his students.

## Tuesday May 5th

A new visitor today, Karen, who drew the curtains and introduced herself as a mental health worker.

'I've heard that you may be going home, and we can arrange follow-up services, by phone of course,' she said. 'Can we have a chat? How are you?'

I stared at her, and thought of everything that had happened. And how, up till now, I had bottled it all up, because my body was so sick. And I didn't want to burden staff – who were looking after my body – with my thoughts. And now I thought my mind was sick. And it all came out. That I didn't see why I should be the only person I knew who had had Coronavirus so badly that I'd ended up in hospital. Why I was the scapegoat. That I had always been the person who

cared for others, that I'd spent years running back and
forth from hospitals, visiting people, sitting by their
sides after operations, taking them to their
appointments. That this had sometimes made me
impatient. That I hadn't cared *enough*. And that when
it came to my turn, there was nobody at my bedside,
ever. That I didn't feel that the people who phoned and
emailed me understood how I felt. That I dreaded
going home as I knew the house and garden would be
in a dreadful state, and that I couldn't cope with any
problems John and Catrin had, or their conditions, or
their medications. That I couldn't cope with anything.
That I dreaded the future. That I loved my bed, my
chair and the ward and the staff, but I didn't feel that I
showed this enough, that I didn't appreciate the staff
enough, that I didn't do everything that they wanted.
That I was ungrateful. That I was not a better person
because of illness. That I had not done anything to
help. That not only had I seen people die, I had seen
them die alone, without their families by their sides –
or able to go to their funerals. That I felt guilty...
Because I was a survivor.

Karen took all this very calmly. I expect she is used to
it. We talked for a while, and then she said she would
arrange for me to have a follow-up service by telephone
when I left, and it would probably be with Conwy
Mind.

It's true I don't feel I have been a better person
because of what I have suffered. So I don't understand

why I had to suffer. I need answers. Both practical and philosophical.

I lay in my bed and looked around. Looking for any form of comfort. Our beds, our chairs, are isolated on the ward. Like islands. The room is a sea, and the ward is an ocean. We are alone in the middle of it.

Felt a bit sniffly, but that might be the beginnings of a slight cold rather than my universal sorrow. A young man in PPE came in and took a swab from the back of my throat.

'You have to test negative before you can go home,' he explained.

Sat thinking about loneliness and isolation. I got out my phone and looked up Matthew Arnold's 'To Marguerite'.

Yes! In the sea of life enisled,
With echoing straits between us thrown,
Dotting the shoreless watery wild,
We mortal millions live alone.
The islands feel their enclasping flow,
And then their endless bounds they know.

But when the moon their hollows lights,
And they are swept by balms of spring,
And in their glens, on starry nights,
The nightingales divinely sing;

And lovely notes, from shore to shore,
Across the sounds and channels pour—

Oh! Then a longing like despair
Is to their furthest channels sent;
For surely, once, they feel, we were
Parts of a single continent!
Now round us spreads the watery plain—

Oh might our marges meet again!
Who order'd that their longing's fire
Should be, as soon as kindled, cool'd?
Who renders vain their deep desire?
A God, a God, their severance ruled!
And bade betwixt their shores to be
The unplumb'd, salt, estranging sea.

In our age, it is the Coronavirus that has separated us
– it is why we all lie in beds distanced from each other,
and indeed from our families.

But no man, and no woman, is an island. We may lie
alone, and separated from our families, but the nurses,
the doctors, the students, the caterers, the cleaners,
the healthcare workers, the therapists – they swim the
'unplumb'd, salt, estranging sea' between our little
islands and bring us food, drink, medication, hope and
company. Our five basic needs.

Yes, there is comfort in this little world, this ocean,
these islands. But then I thought of the great big world

outside – with all its arguments and dissent – which I was going back to, and I shivered.

I then read Arnold's 'Dover Beach', with its plea that we should all love each other, because there is *nothing*. And when I think of the world outside, I don't think that's happening. We are weak and divided, and the virus is strong and united; determined to divide and conquer. And it is not going away.

## Wednesday May 6th

Woke up sniffly, and Susan said I should have an X-ray. I thought I'd be going in a visit in a wheelchair, but instead, two very young and cheerful girls turned up with a huge piece of equipment and did it at my bedside.

I am now addicted to Nutrisips. There is a running sweepstakes on the ward as to the overall favourite flavour. It's strawberry for me, and I start chugging them back straight after breakfast.

Maria had decided today that I should have a shower and wash my hair. She put me into the wheelchair and wheeled me to the bathroom. I can now make it there with a stick, but she wanted me to sit in the chair under the shower while she washed my hair. I didn't feel embarrassed about having no clothes on. You never feel anything like that here; they have seen you at your worst.

Maria had brought in her own hairdryer, as there isn't one in the bathroom. She took my hairbrush and briskly blow-dried my hair; it looks better than it has ever done. Lots of grey though, and needs a cut.

'No hairdressers open,' said Maria, shaking her head, which reminded me of the outside world and its restrictions, which I have tried to forget.

I am in a bubble (more new parlance): a room, a ward, a hospital, a set of people. Outside is a howling wilderness I can't cope with. I haven't watched or listened to the news since I came in. I began to realise for the first time why people moved into sheltered housing and retirement villages, or moved to remote places. To get away from things you can no longer cope with.

I thought I had better get in touch again. I asked Natalie to put the BBC News on the television.

I lay and watched the news in horror. So many thousands dead. So many NHS staff dead, who sacrificed themselves – the photographs of them, in their NHS gear, were heart-breaking. So many thousands of jobs gone with everything closed. So many care home residents dead. People unable to visit their families. People who died without seeing their families. The shortage of proper PPE, and the staff working in hot hospitals smothered in PPE. The bodies piled up in mortuaries. The backlog of funerals. Crematoriums

open seven days a week to deal with the backlog.
Bodies stored in shipping containers and the storage
where they usually put bodies for dissection. Funerals
limited to six, so you couldn't even say goodbye, and
funeral staff in masks and gloves. 1000 people dying
every day. The bosses, millionaires, and billionaires,
who took the opportunity to lay off their staff, and
cheat the furlough scheme. Those selfish people who
broke the rules of the lockdown, while the rest of us
suffered. The lack of testing and of track-and-trace. And
the fact that the UK, one of the richest nations in the
world, is heading for one of the highest death rates.

We had years to prepare for this. Why didn't we
prepare? Why weren't we ready? Why have so many
died? Why didn't we have the PPE ready? And what
will happen if it happens again? Whose fault is this?

But then there were the good news stories. The NHS.
The key workers, the carers, the cleaners, the
caretakers, who carried on as usual. The shop workers,
the delivery drivers, the milkmen, the postmen, the
public services. The people who ran food banks. The
volunteers who kept in touch with the elderly and did
their shopping for them – and just checked that they
were okay.

The Government would call many of these people low-
skilled workers. I don't. They would call many of the
people in this hospital migrant workers. I call them
lifesavers, and I don't care where they came from.

And then there was all the talk of the economy. The thousands now out of work. The thousands who will be out of work as businesses, the performing arts, and hospitality remain closed.

> *As to foreign trade, there needs little to be said. The trading nations of Europe were all afraid of us; no port of France, or Holland, or Spain, or Italy would admit our ships or correspond with us ...* (Defoe)

And so many reports of breaking the lockdown, and of second waves, that I'm not sure that as a nation we have learnt anything. Or realised the virus is not going away.

> *The physicians opposed this thoughtless humour of the people with all their might, and gave out printed directions, spreading them all over the city and suburbs, advising the people to continue reserved, and to use still the utmost caution in their ordinary conduct, notwithstanding the decrease of the distemper, terrifying them with the danger of bringing a relapse upon the whole city, and telling them how such a relapse might be more fatal and dangerous than the whole visitation that had been already ...*
>
> *But it was all to no purpose; the audacious creatures were so possessed with the first joy and so surprised with the satisfaction of seeing a vast decrease in the weekly bills, that they were impenetrable by any new terrors, and would not be persuaded but that the bitterness of death was past; and it was to no more*

*purpose to talk to them than to an east wind; but*
*they opened shops, went about streets, did business,*
*and conversed with anybody that came in their way*
*to converse with, whether with business or without,*
*neither inquiring of their health or so much as being*
*apprehensive of any danger from them, though they*
*knew them not to be sound.*

*This imprudent, rash conduct cost a great many*
*their lives who had with great care and caution*
*shut themselves up and kept retired ...* (Defoe)

## Thursday May 7th

Full round of visits today from everyone. Dr
Mohammed first, beaming, as he told me I had tested
negative and could go home tomorrow. I didn't know
what to say to him. I felt inadequate. I didn't feel
*thank you* was enough.

All followed by Bev and Matt, Physiotherapy, Karen
from Mental Health, Kay the dietician, Claire the
Occupational Therapist, all with leaflets and booklets
for me and promises of follow-up phone calls when I
got home.

After they'd all gone, and I'd said thank you, over and
over, I called John.

'Get me the biggest box of chocolates you can find –
huge – and a massive Thank You card,' I said.

Lay on my bed and sat in my chair. Yasmin drew the curtains so I could have a bit of privacy. I remembered that when I came in, I had thought I had nothing and nobody. Now I have this little space and all these people, and I'm about to lose them again. Love and loss go hand in hand.

And I thought too that I was about to go back into a world where people don't know what it's like to have Coronavirus, and who think it won't happen to them. There would be people who don't see that things are different and will never be the same again. I thought about how the world was divided into two groups: those who have had it and those who have not. I knew what it was like. I had seen those who died. I was the keeper of the secrets. I had power: I knew what it would be like if it happened again. When it happened again.

## Friday May 8th

It isn't as easy leaving hospital as you think, and in fact in the end, it took nearly all day. Something called my Discharge Papers had to be drawn up. The pharmacy had to produce my prescriptions. Lots of telephone calls were made. So I couldn't let John know when he was to fetch me, and of course he can't come into the hospital.

'It's a big thing to leave,' announced Natalie, looking mysterious.

Rosa drew the curtains so I could change back into my own nightie and dressing gown, which had been put into a bag marked Patient Property. I put my phone and hairbrush into my bag. I had nothing else except the toothbrush which Izabella had given me and I took that too. Oh, and I get to keep my stick.

I ended up having breakfast and lunch, which gave me an opportunity to thank Tom, and Jan the cleaner, who came round in the afternoon.

Both Fatima and Maria were in today, and helped me wash and brush my hair.

Everyone seemed so happy that I was going home. Some might say it is because I was bed blocking, that they want people out before the weekend. But I don't think so.

There was a lot of sitting around. My prescription arrived in a plastic bag. Then a huge sheaf of papers, which Natalie put in another bag with all my booklets and leaflets. Then the Ward Clerk, Bethan, who I'd never met, arrived with a list of useful telephone numbers.

Then suddenly it was over.

'You can go as soon as your husband arrives,' announced Natalie, beaming. 'Tell him he can park outside A&E, and to be there in half an hour.'

I wasn't expecting that, and I phoned John, who was as taken aback as I was, and as awkward as I was. He is of the old school. He cannot express emotion, in a time when emotions are running very high indeed. Love in the time of Coronavirus.

He picked up the phone immediately; he must have been waiting.

'I can come home,' I said. 'You can pick me up in half an hour, at the entrance to A&E.' I had to keep the conversation to the bare facts. I had too many conflicting emotions to say anything else. I couldn't say what I felt. I didn't know how I felt.

'I'll be there...' He cleared his throat, tried to say something else, and couldn't. I was coming back from the dead, a changed person. A person with a care plan for body and soul. What do you say? What would you say?

Half an hour later, Natalie came up with a wheelchair.

'It's a bit of a walk, so you'll be better off in this.'

I was sitting in my chair. Fatima and Maria had already stripped the bed and emptied my cupboards. Tom had removed my bed table, and wiped it over. I sat in my chair with my bag and two plastic carriers, as though I had gone already. It was like the last day in the old house.

The three ladies still on the ward waved, and called goodbye and good luck. I was sorry I had not got to know them better, but there was so much coming and going. Different faces every day. Thrown into contact with so many people, with whom you had nothing in common – apart from one thing. And you thought people might die. And you didn't want to get involved in people's lives and problems, because you could barely manage your own. I had wanted to make a friend, but I didn't. I had so little feeling in me, I needed it just to keep going. Just to survive.

It struck me suddenly that it was VE Day. That my mother had welcomed the end of the war, but did not celebrate it because she had lost her father and was still coping with grief. It was over for me too, but I did not feel like celebrating either. She was part of a young generation who helped to rebuild society, and I was part of the old generation coping with the New Normal. It was up to the young to rebuild society. If they could.

Natalie pushed open the two big double doors, seeming curiously excited. I had not been through these doors since I came in.

She wheeled me out onto the long corridor which runs the length of the ward. And all the way along, right down to the exit, it was lined with staff. All of them beaming and clapping. I saw Fatima and Maria, I saw Rosa, Susan and Yasmin. Tom and Qasim, just about to serve tea. Jan the cleaner with his broom. Matt and Beverley from Physio. Claire, Karen, Kay, and Bethan. Nurses and healthcare workers I had never met. The two girls from X-ray. Dr Mohammed at the top, grinning all over his face, with some of his students. All of them applauding.

'I arranged all this!' announced Natalie. 'We always do it when somebody gets better and goes home!'

She wheeled me down to the exit, as I turned from side to side, listening to the applause, and saying thank you, thank you, over and over. I cried, this time tears of joy and gratitude.

And I couldn't help remembering the other scenes – those who had left on trolleys, covered in a white sheet. With no family there to mourn or say their final goodbye. The sacrifices they made.

We went through the Exit doors, and the sound died as they banged behind us. Ward Nine was behind me.

Natalie and I went down in silence to the main entrance. I saw John standing there, looking awkward. I hardly seemed to know him. He came forward, took my hand, and bent down.

'Did you remember the card and chocolates?' were my first words. I had nothing else to say. He was a stranger.

He handed me a large bag.

'It's just starting to rain… you can back the car right up to the doors to put her in,' said Nat.

The beautiful weather was over.

John went out and I gave Natalie the bag.

'Nat, this is for all of you… I wish it were more… I don't know what to… It's …' I stopped. I wanted to hug her and say thank you, but we couldn't. In that moment, I loved her like a daughter. Or a mother. I'm not sure which. Mothers and daughters, carers and the cared for, young and old, were all mixed up in my mind.

'I have to go now,' she said, as John came back in and helped me to my feet. 'Going home.'

'Yes, going home.'

She walked off to the lift, and got in. She didn't look back. There were always other patients. My heart broke. Going home. Leaving home.

John helped me into the car. As we drove off, I turned round and gazed back at the hospital, saying goodbye to all of them. I thought also about what I could do for them… Campaign for better PPE, testing for NHS staff, a pay-rise for all, the writing-off of student nurses' debts. A debt to be repaid. Our debt, not theirs.

John tried to start a conversation.

'Coming home!' he said.

Then, as I didn't reply, he repeated:

'Coming home!'

'Yes,' I said slowly. 'Coming home. Returning.'

I turned my head, away from the hospital, and stared ahead through the front window. I wondered if things would change now. Perhaps, as the planet had been greener and cleaner during lockdown, so it would remain now. Or perhaps we had created a new rod for its back, and people would now drop gloves and masks on the street.

Perhaps we had learned that personal contact spread the virus, and we would give up gathering in pubs, clubs, shops, parks and on beaches. Or perhaps we would not.

Maybe we would learn that a pandemic did not mean a shortage of handwash and toilet rolls in the shops, and we would stop piling our trolleys with pasta and nappies, and fighting over the last bar of soap. Or maybe we would not.

And I wondered if strife and dissent would stop, now that we had all gazed together into the face of Death. If we would realise that there was indeed more that united us than divided us. Or perhaps we hadn't learned, and everything would remain the same. And we would soon, following the examples of our leaders, be at each other's throats again, and all would be forgotten.

*I wish I could say that as the city had a new face, so the manners of the people had a new appearance... but except what of this was to be found in particular families and faces, it must be acknowledged that the general practice of the people was just as it was before, and very little difference was to be seen.*

*Some, indeed, said things were worse; that the morals of the people declined from this very time; that the people, hardened by the danger they had been in, like seamen after a storm is over, were more wicked and more stupid, more bold and hardened, in their vices and immoralities than they were before; but I will not carry it so far neither. It would take up a history of no small length to give a particular of all the gradations by which the course of things in this city came to be restored again, and to run in their own channel as they did before.* (Defoe)

I remember when I was a little girl, I used to ask Mom about the war. What she had done. What it was like working in munitions in a heavily blitzed city. Whether she felt heroic, as though she was living part of history.

She always shrugged.

'Oh, I went from day to day. I just survived,' she said.

And that was my experience. I hadn't learned anything, I hadn't become a better person, I wasn't always as nice to the staff as I should have been, I hadn't tried hard enough, I hadn't pioneered any new medication, I hadn't done anything noble or worthy. Or indeed anything at all. I went from day to day. I just survived. To tell the tale: to warn you. That in the face of death, we are all equal. That we are weak, divided and self-indulgent, and the virus is strong, unified and self-confident. And that time is always running out.

# AFTERWORD

Earlier this year, after nursing a family member diagnosed by telephone as having gastroenteritis, I became ill with symptoms which were not recognised at that time as being those of Coronavirus. I became so ill that I was admitted to hospital, where I tested positive. I then spent nearly three weeks on a ward, separated from all friends and family, with 120 other women and NHS staff who went into battle daily against a faceless enemy.

When I began to recover, I was visited by an Occupational Therapist. There was very little to do on the ward, as books and newspapers were not allowed. She suggested that I kept a diary to keep myself occupied, which I indeed did.

This memoir is based on those diary entries, and though names, dates, and certain details have been changed, everything in it happened. I would also like to add that any medical mistakes in the details of this diary are mine, and I apologise for them. I was an outsider looking in; I was a child trying to make sense of a world I did not understand, and that the grown-ups were too busy to explain to me. Thank you to the medical professionals who helped clarify some of the details in this story, and to Dr Pyrke for his brilliant Foreword; for making sense of what seemed incomprehensible. This is an inadequate tribute to their profession, but I hope what is clear is my heartfelt gratitude.

Upon leaving hospital, I started a course of therapeutic reading while I convalesced. I read Daniel Defoe's *A Journal of the Plague Year*, published in 1722, and was immediately struck with the parallels with our own time. I decided to write my own story.

In fact, Defoe was only five years old at the time of the Great Plague of London. Debate has raged for years as to whether *A Journal of the Plague Year* is a work of fiction or non-fiction, but it seems likely it was based on the journals of his uncle, Henry Foe, who really did live in London during the Great Plague.

This is one of the first personal accounts of life on a ward in the time of Coronavirus, where you are totally cut off from friends and family, as the daily routine of a ward copes with an illness that is simply incurable. It celebrates the bravery of NHS staff and key workers and carers who went into battle every day against a faceless enemy and with inadequate PPE. The doctors who exclaimed in despair, 'We're making this up as we go along,' as they made their endless daily rounds with hundreds of patients, as even more came in on trolleys. The morticians who took bodies away covered with a white sheet because there weren't enough body bags. Catering staff who sat at the bedsides of the very ill, feeding them spoon by spoon. Cleaners who laughed and joked with depressed patients. Nurses who sang to and danced with patients with dementia. Student doctors and nurses who left their studies to join the frontline. Ambulance staff who drove the sick to hospital, cheering up the terrified with jokes. And the patients: those who caught it in the care homes where they worked looking after the old and sick, came into hospital, and asked when they could leave and safely go back to work, 'because we're needed'.

This book was also written in memory of the thousands who died, and continue to die, without any final contact with their loved ones – amongst them, many NHS workers. I wanted to give a voice to the voiceless. This is also their story. They deserve to be remembered. They should not be forgotten.

*Ward Nine: Coronavirus* is a record of these times. It is a story of how the people and NHS staff of Wales reacted to the epidemic; everyday stories of courage in the face of death. It is of course also a love letter to the NHS, to key workers, and carers. It is Wales's story at a certain moment in time. It is our story.

And it's not the end of the story. Convalescing at home for weeks during lockdown, I had numerous follow-up appointments, mainly by telephone – physiotherapy, outpatients', dieticians – all trying to help my body continue its cure.

And then there were those who tried to help cure my mind. I had already had Occupational Therapy in hospital, who referred me to a mental health counsellor. When I left hospital, I was referred to the invaluable Conwy Mind counselling service. I had so much to discuss with them – both personal and general. Why were we not ready for this? Why were we in the situation where bodies were taken away to an overcrowded mortuary, covered in a white sheet as there weren't enough body bags? Why did some make tremendous sacrifices, dying without seeing their families, when others didn't? And what will happen when it happens again? Did we learn anything? Whose fault was it? What can we do? And over and over: why me? How do I cope with having seen people die? How do I ever recover mentally from this? How do I cope with stress and anxiety? How do I return to a New Normal life?

As well as long discussions with my sympathetic counsellor, I embarked on a course of therapeutic reading as listed below – books about sickness and isolation. I realised that I was not alone. None of us are.

The Hearth Centre for the Arts in physical and mental health was the first to recognise and believe in this book, publishing excerpts of the diary in their *Tales of Lockdown* project. For this, I wish to thank them. I would also like to say to all of the women like me – over sixty and still working or seeking work, in essential occupations and in this time of sickness – this book is for you.

And finally, as I have already paid tribute to NHS Wales who cured my body – here I wish to pay tribute to Mind, who cured my soul. This book is a love letter to them both.

# FURTHER READING

These books and poems helped me in my recovery. The first time a plague actually appears in literature is Boccaccio's *Decameron* (1353), in which a group of young people gather to tell tales during an outbreak of the Plague. It's not about the Plague as such, but the point is that stories can help and bring comfort. That they have a beginning, a middle and an end. They bring closure and offer hope.

I read a few futuristic novels in which mankind is often wiped out by a plague or contagion. There are always a few survivors who escape to rebuild the human race. The plague is often a metaphor for some kind of ill in society. I leave it to you to decide what the Coronavirus of our times represents.

Matthew Arnold, 'To Marguerite' (1852) and 'On Dover Beach' (1867)
Albert Camus, *The Plague* (1947)
Daniel Defoe, *A Journal of the Plague Year* (1722)
Betty Macdonald, *The Plague and I* (1948) — An account of a year on a TB ward when tuberculosis was incurable.
Alexander Solzenhitsyn, *Cancer Ward* (1966)

And on isolation, Daniel Defoe's *Robinson Crusoe* (1719) and anything by Anita Brookner and Jean Rhys.

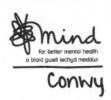

# Conwy

Conwy Mind has been delivering mental health and wellbeing services to the residents of Conwy County since 1985. We offer a range of services to support individuals and families with mild to moderate mental health needs. The support we offer includes:

- Community Hub – Our Community Hub support workers offer a listening ear, training sessions, one to one support and signposting to relevant support services

- Talking Therapies Hub – here we are able to offer counselling, Cognitive Behavioural Therapy and Active Monitoring

- Families Hub – Our Family Support worker offers one to one support, training and signposting for the whole family

- Training Hub – Our trainer is able to provide training sessions in Confidence building, 5 ways to wellbeing and coping with life skills

If you or you know someone who would like to talk to a member of the Conwy Mind team about your/ their mental health, please call us on 01492 879907 or email info@conwymind.org.uk. We are here for you.

For more information about Conwy Mind
please visit www.conwymind.org.uk

Registered Charity Number: 1073596

If you live elsewhere and would like to know more about Mind services near you, as well as mental health information and advice, please visit mind.org.uk